INTERMITTENT FASTING FOR WOMEN

I0424923

+

INTERMITTENT FASTING STARTER COOKBOOK

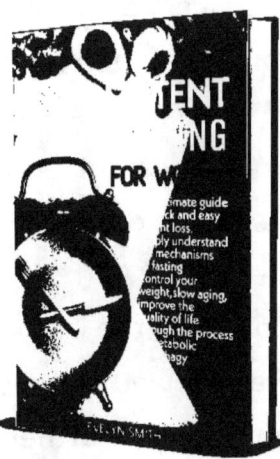 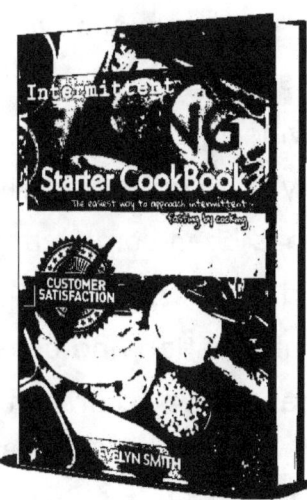

The easiest way to approach intermittent fasting by cooking

Legal & Disclaimer

The information contained in this book and its contents is not designed to replace or take the place of any form of medical or professional advice; and is not meant to replace the need for independent medical, financial, legal or other professional advice or services, as may be required. The content and information in this book has been provided for educational and entertainment purposes only.The content and information contained in this book has been compiled from sources deemed reliable, and it is accurate to the best of the Author's knowledge, information and belief. However, the Author cannot guarantee its accuracy and validity and cannot be held liable for any errors and/or omissions. Further, changes are periodically made to this book as and when needed. Where appropriate and/or necessary, you must consult a professional (including but not limited to your doctor, attorney, financial advisor or such other professional advisor) before using any of the suggested remedies, techniques, or information in this book.Upon using the contents and information contained in this book, you agree to hold harmless the Author from and against any damages, costs, and expenses, including any legal fees potentially resulting from the application of any of the information provided by this book. This disclaimer applies to any loss, damages or injury caused by the use and application, whether directly or indirectly, of any advice or information presented, whether for breach of contract, tort, negligence, personal injury, criminal intent, or under any other cause of action.You agree to accept all risks of using the information presented inside this book.You agree that by continuing to read this book, where appropriate and/or necessary, you shall consult a professional (including but not limited to your doctor, attorney, or financial advisor or such other advisor as needed) before using any of the suggested remedies, techniques, or information in this book.

INTERMITTENT FASTING FOR WOMEN

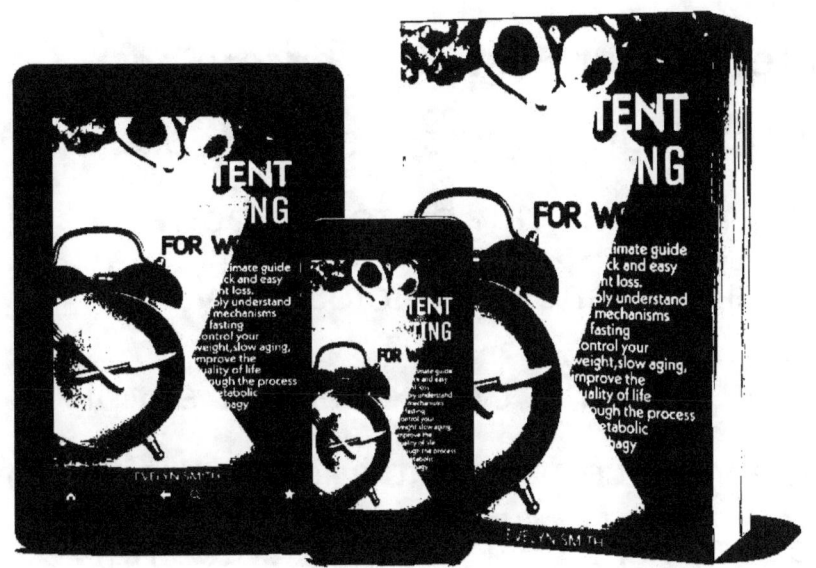

Introduction

A new diet has been introduced for some time: the intermittent fasting diet (also called Intermittent Fasting)

In reality, as we will see better in the course of the article, intermittent fasting is not a real diet but a food program that alternates moments of fasting with intervals on which it is instead allowed to feed.

Intermittent Fasting is becoming increasingly popular as many are the benefits that can be found both physically and psychologically.

Moreover, this type of power supply is also very convenient and practical and adapts very well to our increasingly rapid and frenetic lifestyle.

So if your goal is to lose the extra pounds, then you are in the right place at the right time, because today I will reveal all the details of a truly effective food program proven by various nutritionists.

If you want to learn more then read on below and you will discover the multiple positive effects that you can achieve with the Intermittent Fasting Diet

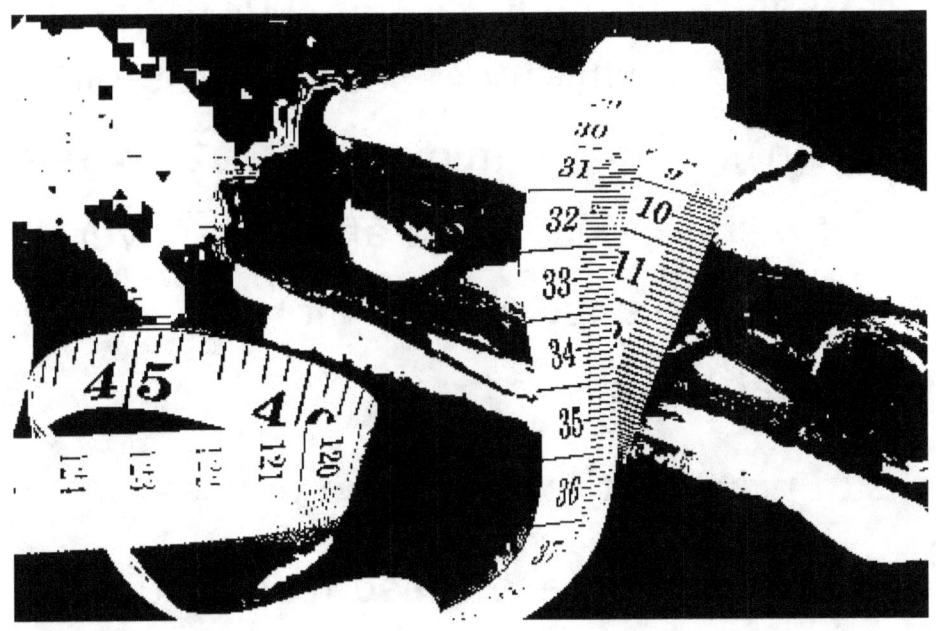

How does intermittent fasting work?

Let's start with the basics ...

What exactly is the diet called "Intermittent Fasting"?

It is a dietary approach in which you will have to enter within the day (or week, depending on the choice you will make when you set the strategic plan), a time of minimum 12-16 hours of fasting, such as to affect the overall caloric balance and hormonal metabolism.

In practice there are two phases:

• a fasting phase called fast, lasting several hours (usually 12 to 20 hours) in which you will not have to introduce any food, except for beverages, such as water, tea, bitter coffee or sugar-free herbal teas

• a phase called fed where you can eat regularly

That's all? That's all.

The Intermittent Fasting is in fact very simple. And that's why it works very well! Soon I'll also explain why.

But first I want to give you some more details.

In fact, there are several methods of intermittent fasting:

1. Intermittent Fasting 16/8: this scheme divides the day into two parts, that is, 8 hours you eat (Fed) and 16

hours of fast (Fast). An example of application is this: skip breakfast and consume the first meal at noon and then don't eat until 20:00.

2. Every other day (5: 2): for two days a week the calorie intake must be reduced to 500-600 calories, while for the rest of the week you can eat what you want. Of course for this type of diet, the days where the calorie intake is reduced must not be consecutive.

3. Eat stop eat: eat once or twice a week from the evening of the day before until dinner the next day.

As you can see, even in this case they are all extremely simple and allow great flexibility

Intermittent Fasting May Affect Men and Women Differently

There is some evidence that intermittent fasting may not be as beneficial for some women as it is for men.

One study showed that blood sugar control actually worsened in women after three weeks of intermittent fasting, which was not the case in men.

There are also many anecdotal stories of women who have experienced changes to their menstrual cycles after starting intermittent fasting.

Such shifts occur because female bodies are extremely sensitive to calorie restriction.

When calorie intake is low — such as from fasting for too long or too frequently — a small part of the brain called the hypothalamus is affected.

This can disrupt the secretion of gonadotropin-releasing hormone (GnRH), a hormone that helps release two reproductive hormones: luteinizing hormone (LH) and follicle stimulating hormone (FSH).

When these hormones cannot communicate with the ovaries, you run the risk of irregular periods, infertility, poor bone health and other health effects .

Although there are no comparable human studies, tests in rats have shown that 3–6 months of alternate-day fasting caused a reduction in ovary size and irregular reproductive cycles in female rats .

For these reasons, women should consider a modified approach to intermittent fasting, such as shorter fasting periods and fewer fasting days.

Intermittent fasting to lose weight:

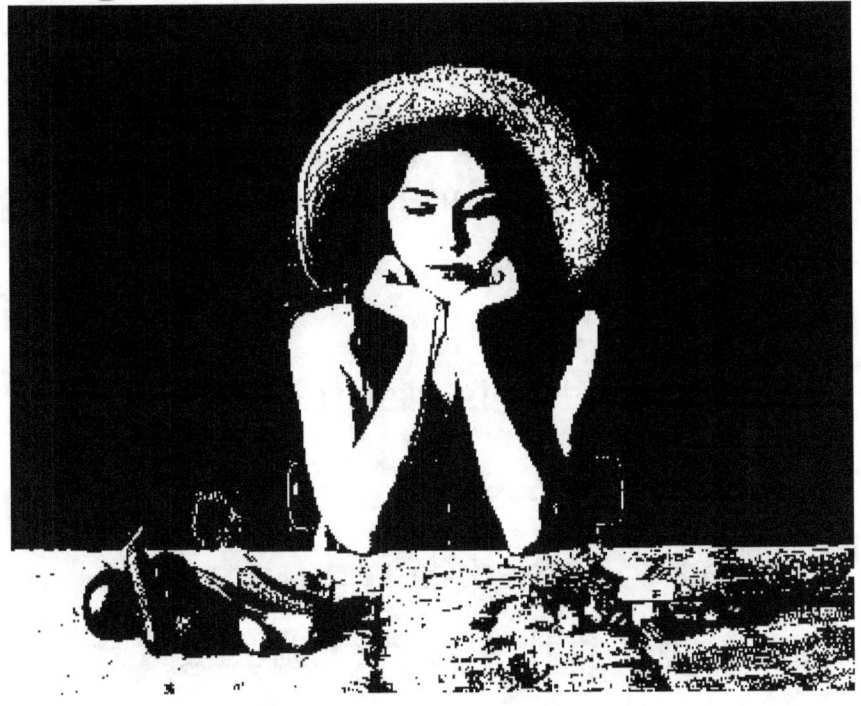

Obviously when we talk about food the first thought goes to the weight and the balance. And therefore to the question: with intermittent fasting is it possible to lose weight?

Absolutely yes! But not only.

If you want to achieve one or all of these three goals:

- Lose weight

- correct various health problems

- live longer

... then this diet is just for you!

In fact it is a great expedient to combine the need to reduce caloric intake and at the same time lighten the effort to give up calories in a natural way.

Having followed many people who wanted to lose weight and who had tried the most varied diets before intermittent fasting, I can say from experience that this methodology is one of those that guarantees the best results.

Not only for the quantity of kilograms lost but above all for the quality of weight loss (very well balanced between lean mass and fat mass) and for ease of weight maintenance once you reach your goal?

How is it possible?

I'll explain why.

There are many people who undertake a diet but very few carry it out. Why do you think? I'll tell you: because it's difficult to give up your favorite foods and because you can't resist the urge to go hungry.

With intermittent fasting, however, both these seemingly insurmountable obstacles are circumvented.

Fasting in fact puts the body in the condition of not having enough energy from food and therefore having to take it from internal reserves (leading to weight loss). Without, however, causing that hunger that we usually feel when we are on a low-calorie diet (reduced in calories).

It seems paradoxical but it is so. Where is the trick?

In the limited duration of fasting.

A prolonged fast in fact demotivates the person, besides putting in place a whole series of compensations from our body, some of which absolutely to be avoided.

While instead fasting only for a limited time makes this practice much easier, because fasting is relatively short and consequently is more bearable.

Other benefits of intermittent fasting

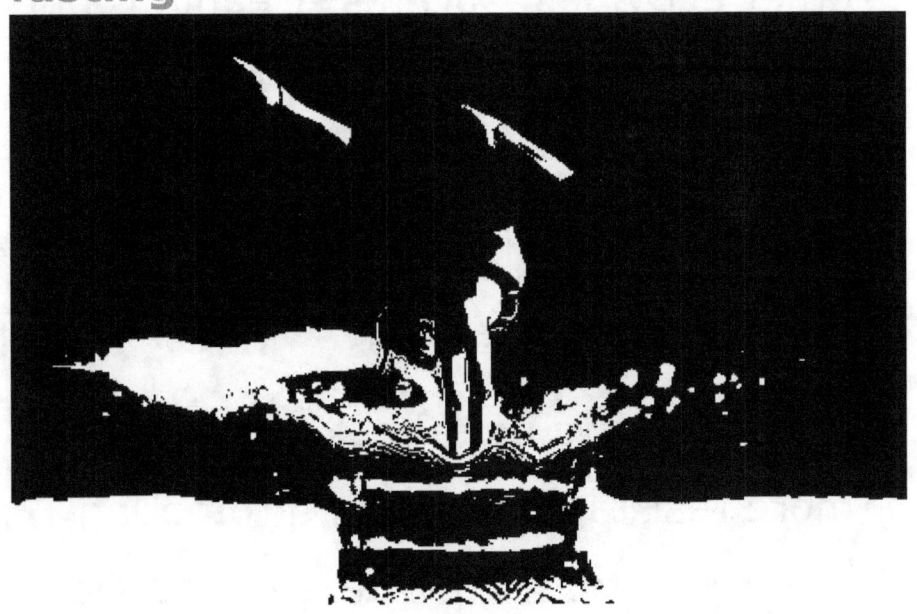

Intermittent Fasting is not only useful for weight loss ... it is a real system to stay healthy for a long time.

In fact, fasting is one of the most powerful means of purifying the body.

When our body is not busy processing food all the time it can devote itself to other activities, such as "cleaning" our body of waste and making many metabolic processes more efficient.

Not to mention the hormonal impact of Intermittent Fasting

Fasting allows us to make our cells more resistant to insulin, promoting protection from important metabolic disorders such as diabetes and the metabolic syndrome.

And finally, during the periods of short fasting, important increases in the production of Growth Hormone have been detected, an important mediator of cell regeneration, useful not only for sportsmen but more generally for all people who wish to slow down the aging process.

How can you guess intermittent fasting is not one of the usual diets that promise miracles in a few weeks.

This is a type of diet that aims to speed up the metabolism and help you lose weight faster by improving cardiovascular health and the immune system in general.

The concept on which it is born is to temporarily disrupt your body and your metabolism, changing the way you usually work your target and forcing it to "wake up" with interesting 360 ° benefits

If you want to undertake this type of diet you will not only lose the extra pounds, but your immune system will become much more resistant to disease.

Many people who have considered this type of diet have felt better physically, and during that time, they felt more energy

Health Benefits of Intermittent Fasting for Women

Intermittent fasting not only benefits your waistline but may also lower your risk of developing a number of chronic diseases.

Heart Health

Heart disease is the leading cause of death worldwide .

High blood pressure, high LDL cholesterol and high triglyceride concentrations are some of the leading risk factors for the development of heart disease.

One study in 16 obese men and women showed intermittent fasting lowered blood pressure by 6% in just eight weeks.

The same study also found that intermittent fasting lowered LDL cholesterol by 25% and triglycerides by 32% .

However, the evidence for the link between intermittent fasting and improved LDL cholesterol and triglyceride levels is not consistent.

A study in 40 normal-weight people found that four weeks of intermittent fasting during the Islamic holiday of Ramadan did not result in a reduction in LDL cholesterol or triglycerides.

Higher-quality studies with more robust methods are needed before researchers can fully understand the effects of intermittent fasting on heart health.

Diabetes

Intermittent fasting may also effectively help manage and reduce your risk of developing diabetes.

Similar to continuous calorie restriction, intermittent fasting appears to reduce some of the risk factors for diabetes.

It does so mainly by lowering insulin levels and reducing insulin resistance.

In a randomized controlled study of more than 100 overweight or obese women, six months of intermittent fasting reduced insulin levels by 29% and insulin resistance by 19%. Blood sugar levels remained the same.

What's more, 8–12 weeks of intermittent fasting has been shown to lower insulin levels by 20–31% and blood sugar levels by 3–6% in individuals with pre-diabetes, a condition in which blood sugar levels are elevated but not high enough to diagnose diabetes .

However, intermittent fasting may not be as beneficial for women as it is for men in terms of blood sugar.

A small study found that blood sugar control worsened for women after 22 days of alternate-day fasting, while there was no adverse effect on blood sugar for men .

Despite this side effect, the reduction in insulin and insulin resistance would still likely reduce the risk of diabetes, particularly for individuals with pre-diabetes.

Weight Loss

Intermittent fasting can be a simple and effective way to lose weight when done properly, as regular short-term fasts can help you consume fewer calories and shed pounds.

A number of studies suggest that intermittent fasting is as effective as traditional calorie-restricted diets for short-term weight loss .

A 2018 review of studies in overweight adults found intermittent fasting led to an average weight loss of 15 lbs (6.8 kg) over the course of 3–12 months.

Another review showed intermittent fasting reduced body weight by 3–8% in overweight or obese adults over a period of 3–24 weeks. The review also found that participants reduced their waist circumference by 3–7% over the same period .

It should be noted that the long-term effects of intermittent fasting on weight loss for women remain to be seen.

In the short term, intermittent fasting seems to aid in weight loss. However, the amount you lose will likely depend on the number of calories you consume during non-fasting periods and how long you adhere to the lifestyle.

It May Help You Eat Less

Switching to intermittent fasting may naturally help you eat less.

One study found that young men ate 650 fewer calories per day when their food intake was restricted to a four-hour window .

Another study in 24 healthy men and women looked at the effects of a long, 36-hour fast on eating habits. Despite consuming extra calories on the post-fast day, participants dropped their total calorie balance by 1,900 calories, a significant reduction .

Other Health Benefits

A number of human and animal studies suggest that intermittent fasting may also yield other health benefits.

Reduced inflammation: Some studies show that intermittent fasting can reduce key markers of inflammation.

Chronic inflammation can lead to weight gain and various health problems .

Improved psychological well-being: One study found that eight weeks of intermittent fasting decreased depression and binge eating behaviors while improving body image in obese adults .

Increased longevity: Intermittent fasting has been shown to extend lifespan in rats and mice by 33–83%. The effects on longevity in humans is yet to be determined .

Preserve muscle mass: Intermittent fasting appears to be more effective at retaining muscle mass compared to continuous calorie restriction. Higher muscle mass helps you burn more calories, even at rest.

Specifically, the health benefits of intermittent fasting for women need to be studied more extensively in well-designed human studies before any conclusions can be drawn .

Frequently Asked Questions
Here are answers to the most common questions about intermittent fasting.

1. Can I Drink Liquids During the Fast?

Yes. Water, coffee, tea and other non-caloric beverages are fine. Do not add sugar to your coffee. Small amounts of milk or cream may be okay.

Coffee can be particularly beneficial during a fast, as it can blunt hunger.

2. Isn't It Unhealthy to Skip Breakfast?

No. The problem is that most stereotypical breakfast skippers have unhealthy lifestyles. If you make sure to eat healthy food for the rest of the day then the practice is perfectly healthy.

3. Can I Take Supplements While Fasting?

Yes. However, keep in mind that some supplements like fat-soluble vitamins may work better when taken with meals.

4. Can I Work out While Fasted?

Yes, fasted workouts are fine. Some people recommend taking branched-chain amino acids (BCAAs) before a fasted workout.

You can find many BCAA products on Amazon.

5. Will Fasting Cause Muscle Loss?

All weight loss methods can cause muscle loss, which is why it's important to lift weights and keep your protein intake high. One study showed that intermittent fasting causes less muscle loss than regular calorie restriction (16Trusted Source).

6. Will Fasting Slow Down My Metabolism?

No. Studies show that short-term fasts actually boost metabolism (14Trusted Source, 15Trusted Source). However, longer fasts of 3 or more days can suppress metabolism (36Trusted Source).

7. Should Kids Fast?

Allowing your child to fast is probably a bad idea.

Does intermittent fasting work?

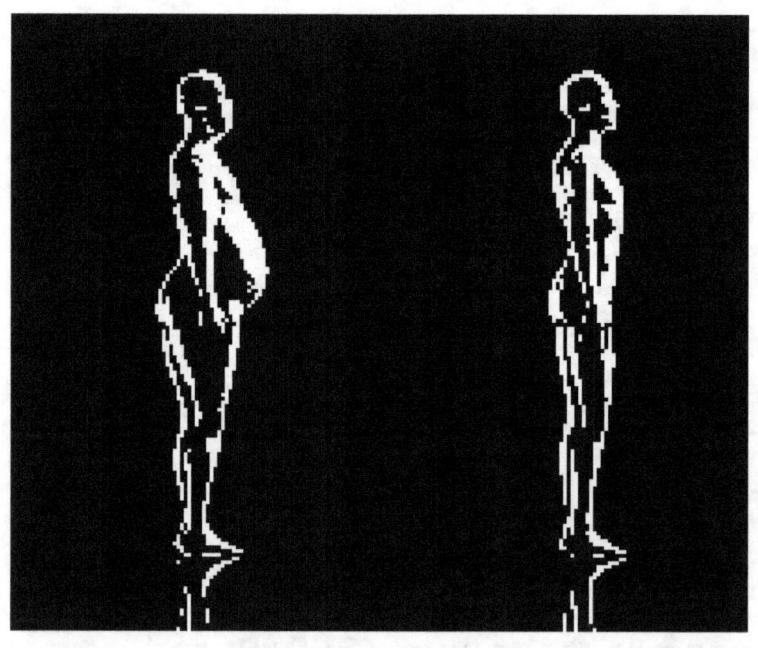

We hear about fasting since ancient times. Many peoples of the world have practiced fasting for purifying, healthy and religious reasons.

And in fact the origins of fasting are lost in the mists of time.

Many even claim that fasting is the "normal mode of functioning of the human being". In fact, if you think about it, over the millennia there has never been such availability of food as it is today.

Therefore the man of the past, for hundreds of thousands of years, has always fasted.

He almost always fasted, at least until the hunters of the tribe could not hunt some big animal, thus giving the possibility to all the various families to take refreshment and "fill up with food"

This phenomenon has happened for a very long time. It is practically inherent in our DNA.

In a world characterized by scarcity of food, the interval of fasting periods more or less long and periods of "binge eating" is practically normal.

This is exactly why intermittent fasting works.

In fact, with the intermittent fasting diet, you introduce nutrients in a cyclic way (the two phases that alternate) and this is a good thing since this regime respects the physiology of the human body.

So, when asked, intermittent fasting works, the answer is certainly yes.

This is a powerful tool that, once you understand how it works, will help you lose excess weight, maintain a healthy weight, live longer and get rid of many diseases.

Types of Intermittent Fasting

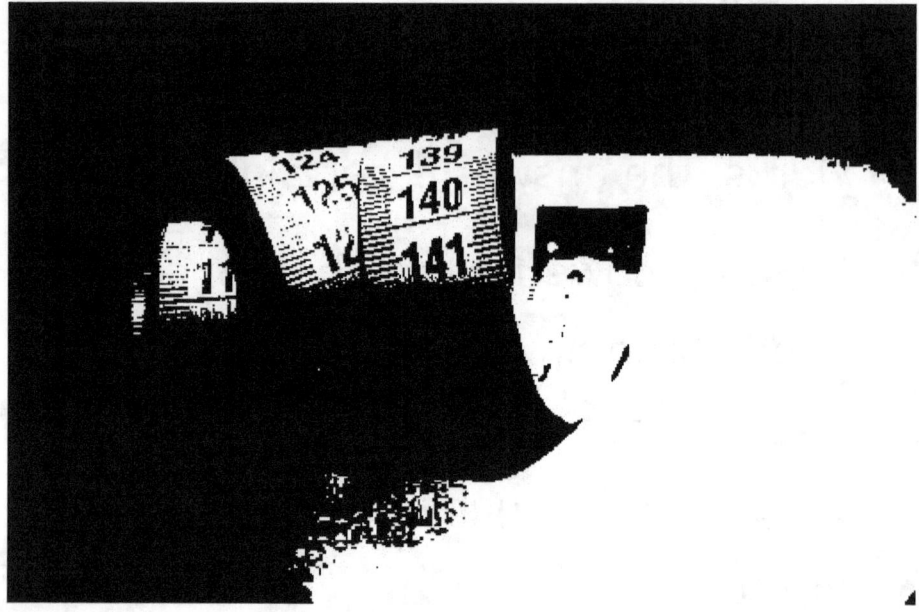

The following are the most popular examples of intermittent fasting and can be adapted as needed. In the Intermittent Fasting Guide you will find an in-depth look at each of the types of fasting listed, which can be associated with a sport.

Diet LeanGains or Intermittent Fasting 16: 8

The LeanGains diet or intermittent fasting 16: 8 provides a feeding window - feeding window - of 8 hours followed by 16 hours of fasting. In the most basic version, we essentially skip breakfast.

Intermittent Fasting 18: 6

Similar to the LeanGains diet. Here the feeding window is 6 hours and fasting for 8 hours.

Fast or 5: 2 diet

For 5 days a week we eat in a classic way. In the remaining two, around 500 calories are consumed.

Warrior Diet or Warrior Diet

The feeding window is 4 hours, usually for dinner. In the rest of the day you can choose to consume fresh vegetables and light fruit.

Alternating Fasting or Alternating-day Fasting

A day of fasting alternates with a day when food is consumed. The day you eat you can choose to do it all day or in a specific feeding window.

OMAD diet

The OMAD diet - One Meal A Day - includes a feeding window of 1 hour a day and 23 hours of fasting. In practice, a full meal a day.

Complete fasting

Once a week or when you want to fast for a whole day. On other days you can choose whether to follow intermittent fasting or not. It is also possible to fast more

lunch, as for example for 5 days.

Best Types of Intermittent Fasting for Women

When it comes to dieting, there is no one-size-fits-all approach. This also applies to intermittent fasting.

Generally speaking, women should take a more relaxed approach to fasting than men.

This may include shorter fasting periods, fewer fasting days and/or consuming a small number of calories on the fasting days.

Here are some of the best types of intermittent fasting for women

Crescendo Method: Fasting 12–16 hours for two to three days a week. Fasting days should be nonconsecutive and spaced evenly across the week (for example, Monday, Wednesday and Friday).

Eat-stop-eat (also called the 24-hour protocol): A 24-hour full fast once or twice a week (maximum of two times a week for women). Start with 14–16 hour fasts and gradually build up.

The 5:2 Diet (also called "The Fast Diet"): Restrict calories to 25% of your usual intake (about 500 calories) for two days a week and eat "normally" the other five days. Allow one day between fasting days.

Modified Alternate-Day Fasting: Fasting every other day but eating "normally" on non-fasting days. You are allowed to consume 20–25% of your usual calorie intake (about 500 calories) on a fasting day.

The 16/8 Method (also called the "Leangains method"): Fasting for 16 hours a day and eating all calories within an eight-hour window. Women are advised to start with 14-hour fasts and eventually build up to 16 hours.

Whichever you choose, it is still important to eat well during the non-fasting periods. If you eat a large amount of unhealthy, calorie-dense foods during the non-fasting periods, you may not experience the same weight loss and health benefits.

At the end of the day, the best approach is one that you can tolerate and sustain in the long-term, and which does not result in any negative health consequences.

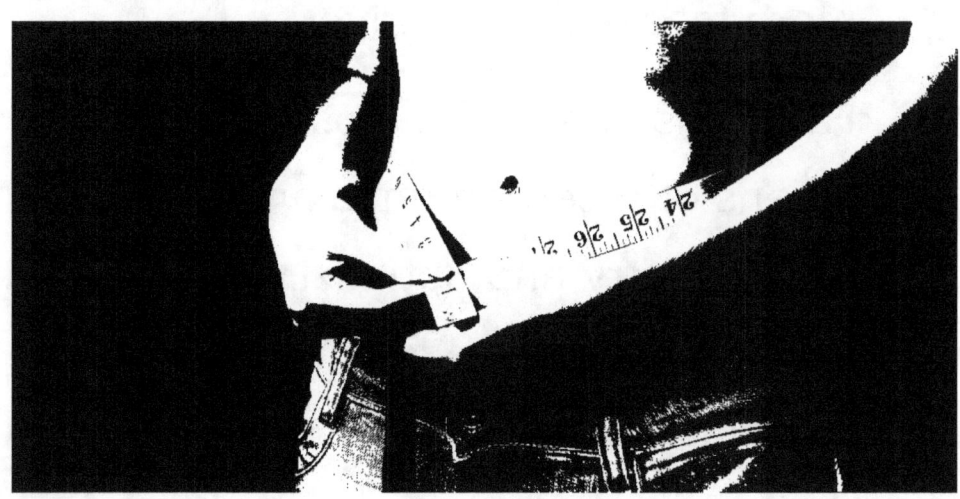

Easier fasting

Yes, because in reality very few people are endowed with the momentum and willpower needed to face a fast that can last up to several days.

Hence the desire for a simpler and more feasible alternative ...

Fasting is one of the most powerful means of resetting unbalanced biochemistry and optimizing conditions that can lead to life extension. But for many people it is difficult to implement, especially for two reasons ...

How is intermittent fasting easier?

Two of the main reasons why prolonged fasting is difficult to implement are the following.

First of all it would be appropriate to take the time dedicated to a prolonged depurative ritual. Then it is advised to set up also the best conditions to operate a fast (to be followed by a nutritionist or by the doctor, to be able to remain focused on this goal, etc.) given the effort required to complete it (it is useless to deny it).

In short, putting a prolonged fasting into practice decidedly difficult makes it difficult if not impossible for many people to approach this healthy practice.

At most, many well-intentioned people simply read something about fasting, try, then get upset and give up and don't try anymore ...

But thanks to intermittent fasting the practice of abstaining from food (and calories in general) becomes decidedly easier for everyone to implement.

Also because unlike prolonged fasting, which may require an interruption of the most demanding activities, intermittent fasting takes advantage of daily tasks

Distract yourself and fast

In what sense does it "take advantage of daily commitments"? pulling a single day without eating can be even easier to bear if you are immersed in your usual activities in the meantime.

So with intermittent fasting there is no need to change anything of one's daily activity rituals. Indeed these can just distract the mind from the thought of food.

A brief workout such as functional training or 30-45 minute yoga on the day of this short fast would even be recommended.

Finally, with a minimum of good will, anyone can FAST and gain health and fitness without necessarily having the mental strength of a fakir.

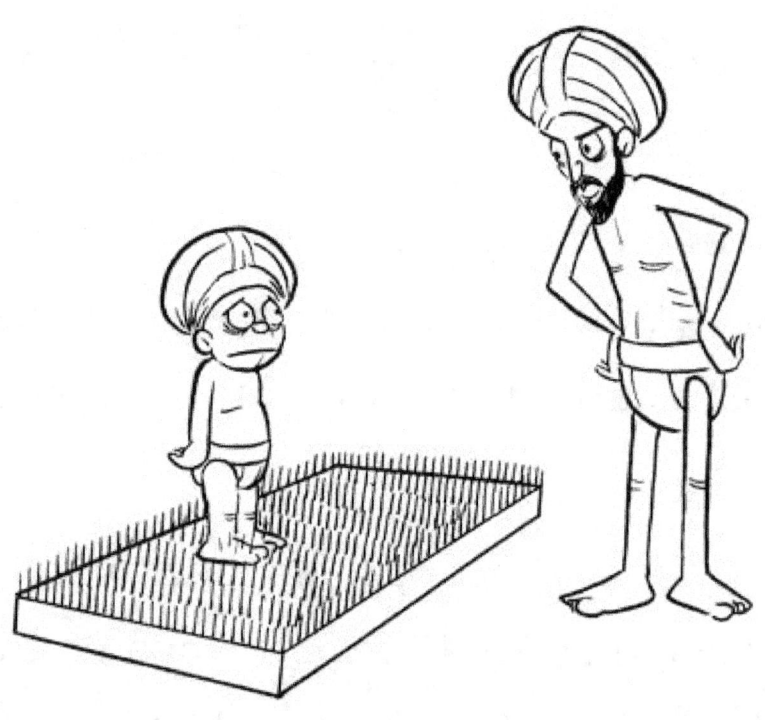

Another grandiose element of intermittent fasting that facilitates its implementation concerns the fact that it is relatively elastic in its duration. That is, the time to devote to fasting is relatively short, therefore bearable

Characteristics of intermittent fasting

Intermittent fasting is an extremely natural way of eating.

During its evolution, the complex and refined metabolism of the human being was forged by an innumerable series of intermittent fasts, not binge eating!

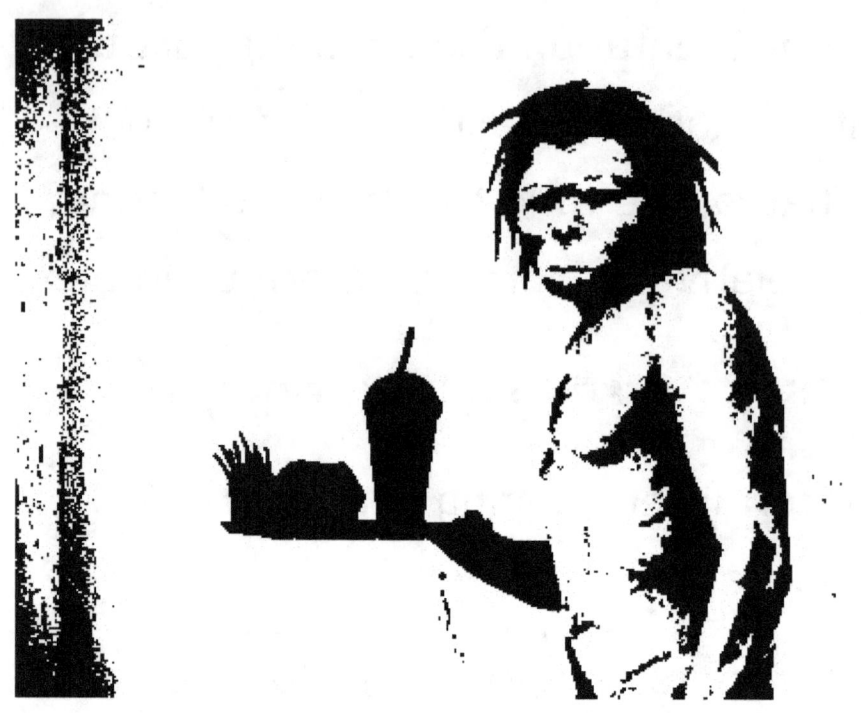

If you think about the difficulty of getting nourishment in nature you can guess that the body has all the means to survive days and days with little or nothing.

Our body is perfectly designed to pass through more or less long periods of absence of food. Not only can it do but it is also a prerogative for its optimal functioning.

It is more normal for us to fast intermittently than to eat 3 or 4 times a day. That is to say, the unhealthy deviation consists precisely in feeding too much, so the remedy is to return to the natural rhythms of intermittent fasting.

Religious fasting

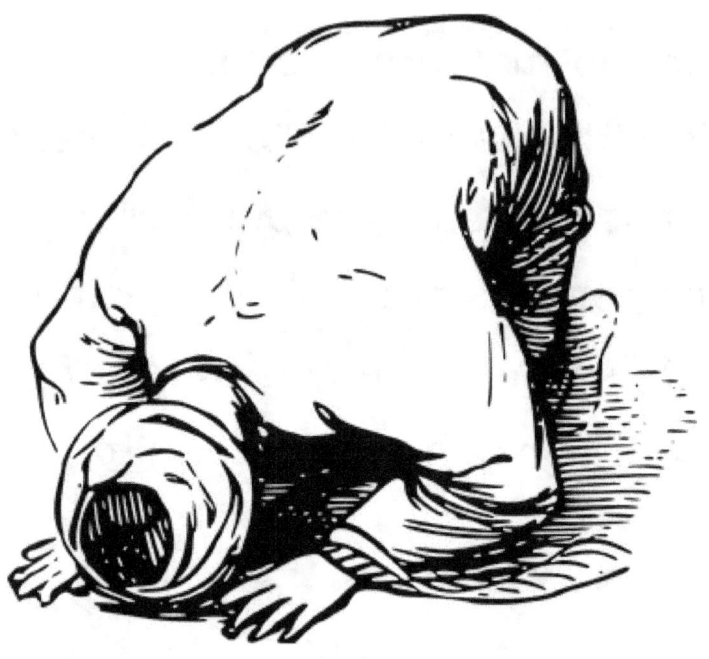

Furthermore, in the course of our most recent evolution, intermittent fasting has continued to be present and widespread for religious reasons. In many different religions and rituals around the world the need has always been felt to devote periods of time to abstaining from food.

Voluntary abstention from food is a form of self-discipline that increases the perception of control that our mind can have on the body. Unleashed desires often cause unhappiness that lasts long after the brief enjoyment of their immediate satisfaction

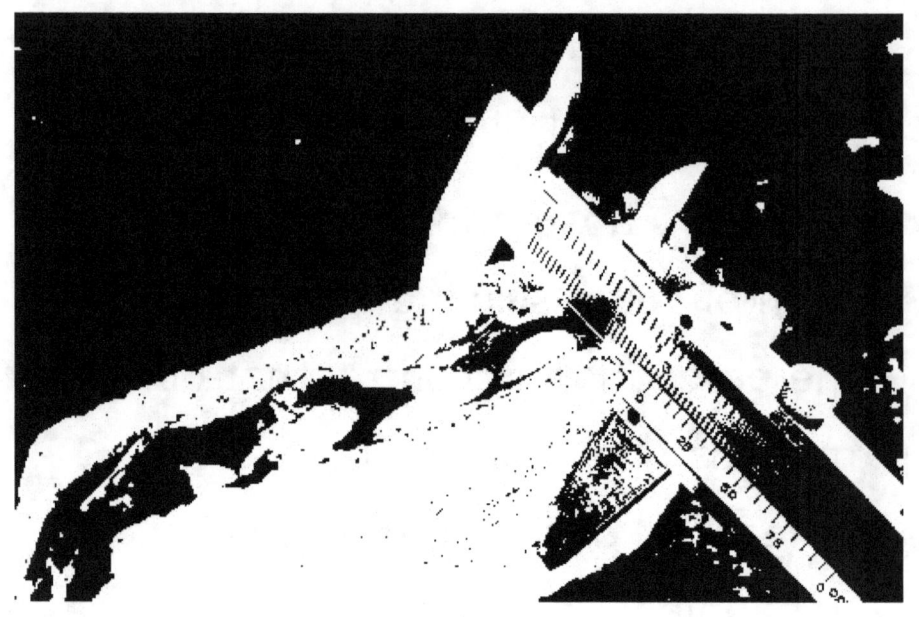

A certain inner solidity due to the fact of "taking back the bridles" of our behavior is associated with greater happiness. This is probably why religions often prescribe programmed food waivers.

Certainly today numerous researches confirm that the metabolic rest that can be implemented with intermittent fasting is one of the most effective and easy to implement ways to get better and live longer

4 ways in which intermittent fasting changes metabolism.

When you stop taking calories for enough time in your body, certain cellular and molecular changes occur ...

1) Activation of autophagy

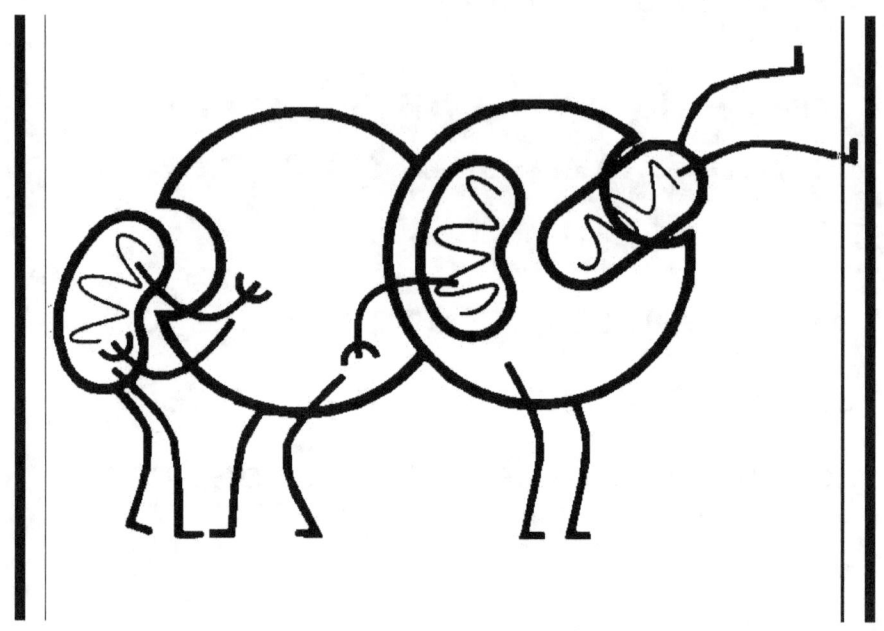

One of the most important events
taking place in a fasting organism is
autophagy1,2. The intelligence of the
body under the stimulus of lack of

energy from food sources (during fasting) begins to exploit damaged cells and molecules to feed themselves.

The body thus begins to sustain itself thanks to the use of some of its components now aged and therefore to be replaced. Autophagy in this way expresses two benefits in one: it supplies new energy to the body and at the same time eliminates certain parts that are now dysfunctional.

... AND CELL REGENERATION

Following the elimination of damaged components the body is induced to synthesize new ones. The newly generated components (cells, proteins, etc.) will be healthier than the previous ones because they are just "churned out" by the body's biosynthetic system.

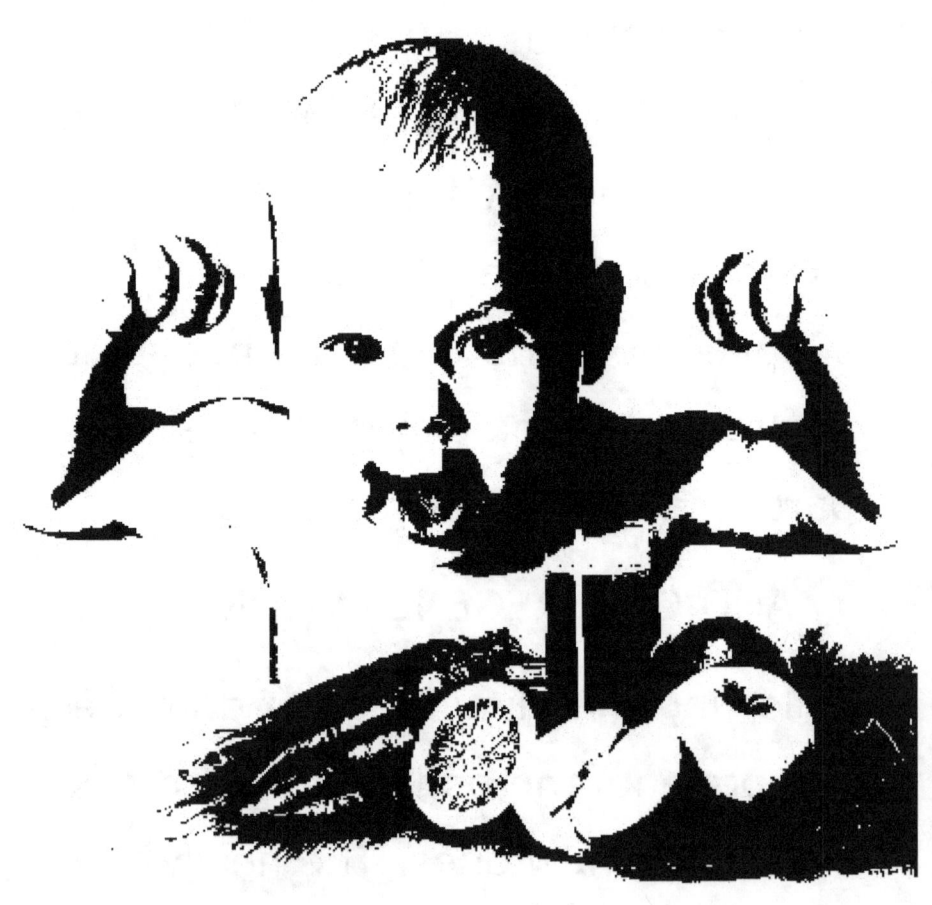

Whenever this cycle of elimination and regeneration occurs, the body is partly renewed and renewed, prolonging its longevity potential.

Not bad...

With a simple short (intermittent) fast the body renews itself.

We had already encountered this process in the practice of the fasting diet. Certainly, however, this last approach is definitely more challenging because it lasts 5 days. On the contrary, an intermittent fasting lasts only from 16 to 24 hours (including the hours of natural night fasting).

2) Synthesis of the GH hormone

GH is the acronym of Growth Hormone, that is growth hormone.

This hormone simultaneously activates the development of muscle mass and the loss of body fat3. Two important benefits for maintaining a lean and healthy body.

The body tends to produce less GH over the years during the aging process. Fasting makes it possible to give a new boost to the production of this important hormone4,5 in a completely natural way

3)Profilo insulinico

With intermittent fasting the insulin sensitivity improves and consequently the average insulin levels are lowered. This allows easier access to the use of deposited fat reserves

3) Insulin profile

During an intermittent fasting practice several protective action genes are activated. In particular, protective genes are activated against different pathologies7 and genes closely involved in the mechanisms of longevity

The 5 Benefits of Intermittent Fasting
1) Weight Loss

Intermittent fasting is truly a powerful way to reduce excess fat. Its action on specific hormones such as GH, insulin and noradrenaline makes it an effective tool to reduce abdominal inflammatory fat (see article on belly fat).

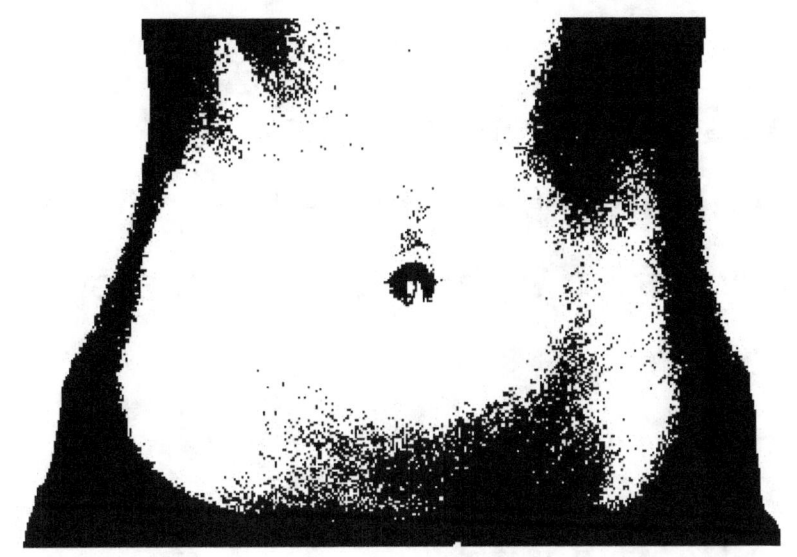

Moreover, even the calorie reduction in the strict sense that occurs during intermittent fasting contributes to weight

2) Anti-inflammatory effect

Several studies show that fasting reduces the inflammatory state of the body9,10.

This leads to a consequent benefit against numerous chronic degenerative pathologies that develop starting from a chronic inflammatory condition.

3) Heart health

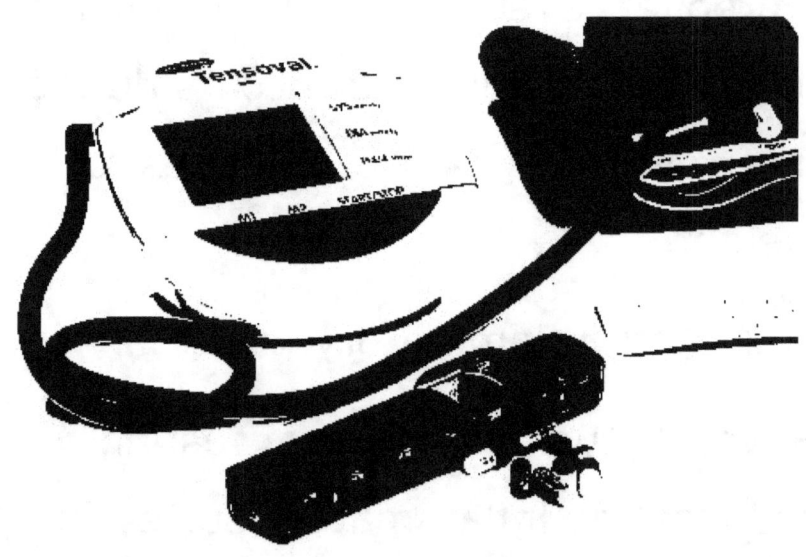

A series of benefits of intermittent fasting linked to heart health 11

makes it particularly suitable for maintaining the cardiovascular system in perfect condition.

Specifically, intermittent fasting can reduce inflammation, blood sugars (improve insulin sensitivity), triglycerides and "bad" LDL cholesterol. All this produces a synergy that promotes the health of the heart and arteries

#4) Antitumor protection

Several studies show a correlation between intermittent fasting and special protection against cancer cells12,13. By now it is becoming increasingly clear how reducing the quantity and frequency of meals can protect better than any other defense against the development of "mad cells"

#5) Maintenance and optimization of brain and nerve functions

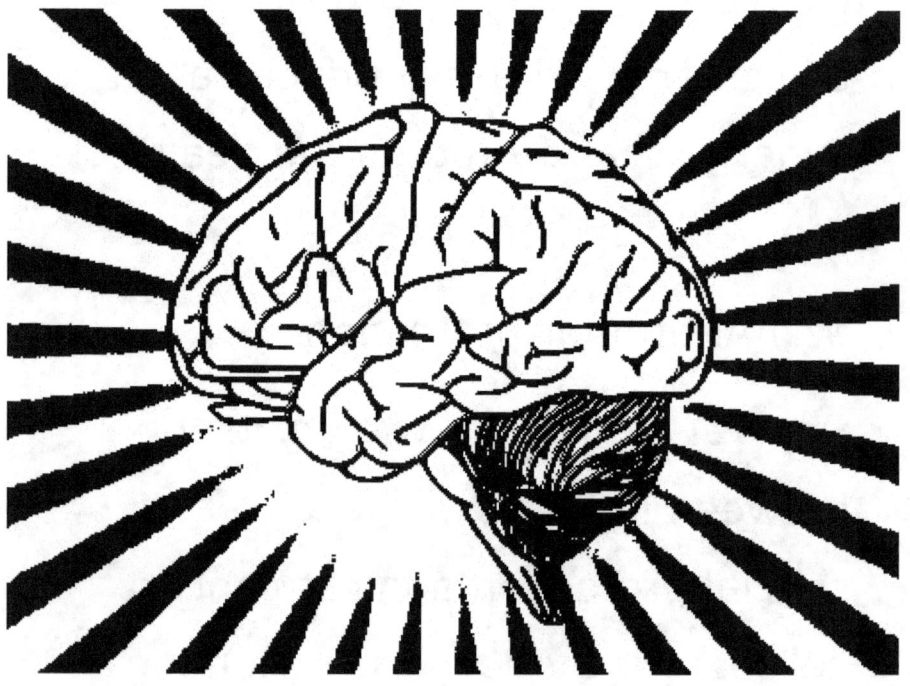

This benefit of intermittent fasting is associated with its general anti-aging effect but is also expressed markedly in relation to neurons.

Some studies show that intermittently fasting stimulates the processes of nerve regeneration15 (postnatal neurogenesis). It also protects against neurodegenerative diseases16.17 and against Alzheimer's disease18.

AND AN ADDITIONAL BENEFIT ...

To this list of 5 points that you have just seen, I would also add another very useful side benefit ... increase your willpower. Willpower is like a muscle that increases its power with training.

More willpower means greater self-control in our lives. A wise and nonviolent self-control helps to direct our lives constructively and thus leads us to a greater good

How intermittent fasting works

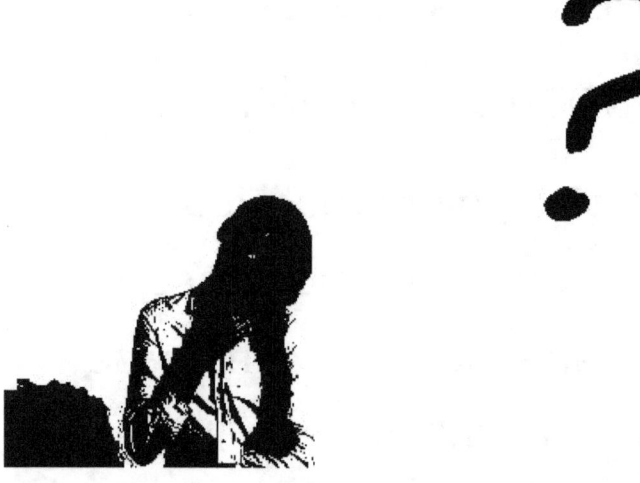

Intermittent fasting is nothing exotic ... who knows how many times you

have already put it into practice without knowing it.

Maybe because of the haste and the little time available you missed the breakfast arriving until lunchtime without taking calories of any kind. This is a classic example of intermittent "unconscious" fasting.

One of the most beautiful things that make intermittent fasting easy to follow even for the less "aggressive" is that you can take advantage of the hours of sleep. The hours of sleep are counted in the minimum 16 hours of fasting.

To begin the practice of intermittent fasting you can easily dine and then no longer touch food or calories of any kind until lunchtime the next day.

Indeed...

The time range for caloric abstention is from 16 to 24 hours (uninterrupted). A short time, especially if you think that in this count the hours of sleep are already included.

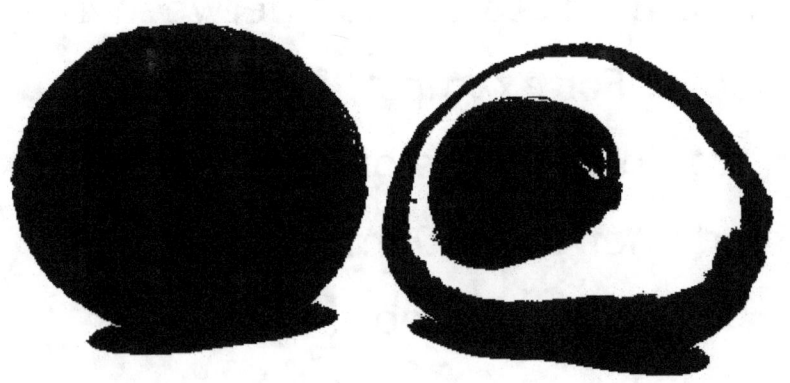

Intermittent fasting easy version
Duration: 16 hours (including overnight fasting).

Mode: starts with dinner, say at 8.00pm. For example, if you finish dinner at 20:30. From that moment on, no food is touched until 12:30 on the following day.

Intermittent fasting Intermediate version

Of course you can decide to make any intermediate version between 16-24 hours. For example, let's say you want to do 18 hours of fasting and finish dinner at 8.30pm ... in this case, don't touch food until 2.30pm the following day.

Intermittent fasting difficult version

Duration: 24 hours (including overnight fasting)

Mode: starts with breakfast for example at 7:00, which you will have finished say at 7:30. Then the intake of calories is interrupted throughout the day and night until breakfast the following day at 7:00.

10 Myths About Fasting and Meal Frequency

Fasting has become increasingly common.

In fact, intermittent fasting, a dietary pattern that cycles between periods of fasting and eating, is often promoted as a miracle diet.

Yet, not everything you've heard about meal frequency and your health is true.

Here are 10 myths about fasting and meal frequency.

1. Skipping breakfast makes you fat

One ongoing myth is that breakfast is the most important meal of the day.

People commonly believe that skipping breakfast leads to excessive hunger, cravings, and weight gain.

One 16-week study in 283 adults with overweight and obesity observed no weight difference between those who ate breakfast and those who didn't .

Thus, breakfast doesn't largely affect your weight, although there may be some individual variability. Some studies even suggest that people who lose weight over the long term tend to eat breakfast .

What's more, children and teenagers who eat breakfast tend to perform better at school .

As such, it's important to pay attention to your specifc needs. Breakfast is beneficial for some people, while others can skip it without any negative consequences.

2. Eating frequently helps reduce hunger

Some people believe that periodic eating helps prevent cravings and excessive hunger.

Yet, the evidence is mixed.

Although some studies suggest that eating more frequent meals leads to reduced hunger, other studies have found no effect or even increased hunger levels .

One study that compared eating three or six high-protein meals per day found that eating three meals reduced hunger more effectively.

That said, responses may depend on the individual. If frequent eating reduces your cravings, it's probably a good idea. Still, there's no evidence that snacking or eating more often reduces hunger for everyone.

3. Eating frequently boosts your metabolism

Many people believe that eating more meals increases your metabolic rate, causing your body to burn more calories overall.

Your body indeed expends some calories digesting meals. This is termed the thermic effect of food TEF.

On average, TEF uses around 10% of your total calorie intake.

However, what matters is the total number of calories you consume — not how many meals you eat.

Eating six 500-calorie meals has the same effect as eating three 1,000-calorie meals. Given an average TEF of 10%, you'll burn 300 calories in both cases.

Numerous studies demonstrate that increasing or decreasing meal frequency does not affect total calories burned

4. Your brain needs a regular supply of dietary glucose

Some people claim that if you don't eat carbs every few hours, your brain will stop functioning.

This is based on the belief that your brain can only use glucose for fuel.

However, your body can easily produce the glucose it needs via a process called gluconeogenesis .

Even during long-term fasting, starvation, or very very-low-carb diets, your body can produce ketone bodies from dietary fats .

Ketone bodies can feed parts of your brain, reducing its glucose requirement significantly.

However, some people report feeling fatigued or shaky when they don't eat for a while. If this applies to you, you should consider keeping snacks on hand or eating more frequently

5. Frequent meals can help you lose weight

Since eating more frequently doesn't boost your metabolism, it likewise doesn't have any effect on weight loss

.

Indeed, a study in 16 adults with obesity compared the effects of eating 3 and 6 meals per day and found no difference in weight, fat loss, or appetite .

Some people claim that eating often makes it harder for them to adhere to a healthy diet. However, if you find that eating more often makes it easier for you to eat fewer calories and less junk food, feel free to stick with it.

6. Fasting puts your body in starvation mode

One common argument against intermittent fasting is that it puts your body into starvation mode, thus shutting down your metabolism and preventing you from burning fat.

While it's true that long-term weight loss can reduce the number of calories you burn over time, this happens no matter what weight loss method you use .

There's no evidence that intermittent fasting causes a greater reduction in calories burned than other weight loss strategies.

In fact, short-term fasts may increase your metabolic rate.

This is due to a drastic increase in blood levels of norepinephrine, which stimulates your metabolism and instructs your fat cells to break down body fat.

Studies reveal that fasting for up to 48 hours can boost metabolism by 3.6–14%. However, if you fast much longer, the effects can reverse, decreasing your metabolism.

One study showed that fasting every other day for 22 days did not lead to a reduction in metabolic rate but a 4% loss of fat mass, on average.

7. Your body can only use a certain amount of protein per meal

Some people claim that you can only digest 30 grams of protein per meal and that you should eat every 2–3 hours to maximize muscle gain.

However, this is not supported by science.

Studies show that eating your protein in more frequent doses does not affect muscle mass.

The most important factor for most people is the total amount of protein consumed — not the number of meals it's spread over.

8. Intermittent fasting makes you lose muscle

Some people believe that when you fast, your body starts burning muscle for fuel.

Although this happens with dieting in general, no evidence suggests that it occurs more with intermittent fasting than other methods.

On the other hand, studies indicate that intermittent fasting is better for maintaining muscle mass.

In one review, intermittent fasting caused a similar amount of weight loss as continuous calorie restriction — but with much less reduction in muscle mass .

Another study showed a modest increase in muscle mass for people who consumed all their calories during one huge meal in the evening.

Notably, intermittent fasting is popular among many bodybuilders, who find that it helps maintain muscle alongside a low body fat percentage.

9. Intermittent fasting is bad for your health

While you may have heard rumors that intermittent fasting harms your health, studies reveal that it has several impressive health benefits .

For example, it changes your gene expression related to longevity and immunity and has been shown to prolong lifespan in animals.

It also has major benefits for metabolic health, such as improved insulin sensitivity and reduced oxidative stress, inflammation, and heart disease risk.

It may also boost brain health by elevating levels of brain-derived neurotrophic factor (BDNF), a hormone that may protect against depression and various other mental conditions

10. Intermittent fasting makes you overeat

Some individuals claim that intermittent fasting causes you to overeat during the eating periods.

While it's true that you may compensate for calories lost during a fast by automatically eating a little more afterward, this compensation isn't complete.

One study showed that people who fasted for 24 hours only ended up eating about 500 extra calories the next day — far fewer than the 2,400 calories they'd missed during the fat.Because it reduces overall food intake and insulin levels while boosting metabolism, norepinephrine levels, and human growth hormone (HGH) levels, intermittent fasting makes you lose fat — not gain it.According to one review, fasting for

3–24 weeks caused average weight and belly fat losses of 3–8% and 4–7%, respectively.

As such, intermittent fasting may be one of the most powerful tools to lose weight

What you can drink during intermittent fasting

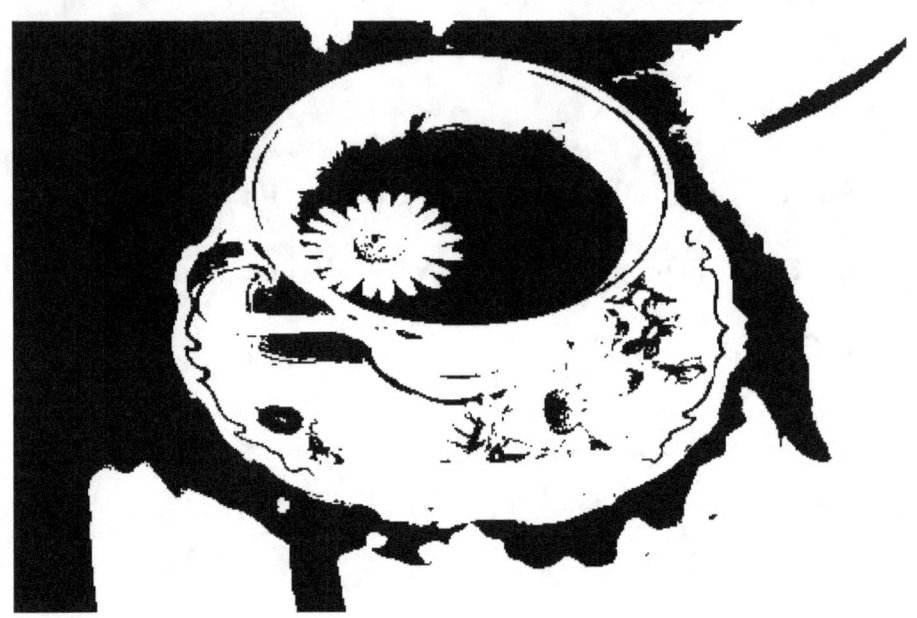

You can drink it at will, indeed it is advisable. Also because good hydration accelerates the metabolism and reduces the sense of hunger. But not all drinks are good for this type of fasting.

The allowed drinks are (without sugar or sweeteners):

Water (possibly in a glass bottle or filtered with an active carbon filter)

Herbal tea (with water not from the tap)

Coffee

You

However, herbal teas, coffee and tea should not be sweetened with sweeteners containing sugar. If you can't do without it you can use some stevia to sweeten without calories and naturally.

The 6 Best Teas to Lose Weight and Belly Fat

Tea is a beverage enjoyed around the world.

You can make it by pouring hot water onto tea leaves and allowing them to steep for several minutes so their flavor infuses into the water.

This aromatic beverage is most commonly made from the leaves of Camellia sinensis, a type of evergreen shrub native to Asia.

Drinking tea has been associated with many health benefits, including protecting cells from damage and reducing the risk of heart disease

Some studies have even found that tea may enhance weight loss and help fight belly fat. Certain types have been found to be more effective than others at achieving this.

Below are six of the best teas for increasing weight loss and decreasing body fat.

1. Green Tea

Green tea is one of the most well-known types of tea, and is linked with many health benefits.

It's also one of the most effective teas for weight loss. There is substantial evidence linking green tea to decreases in both weight and body fat.

In one 2008 study, 60 obese people followed a standardized diet for 12 weeks while regularly drinking either green tea or a placebo.

Over the course of the study, those who drank green tea lost 7.3 pounds (3.3 kg) more weight than the placebo group .

Another study found that people who consumed green tea extract for 12 weeks experienced significant decreases in body weight, body fat and waist circumference, compared to a control group .

This may be because green tea extract is especially high in catechins, naturally occurring antioxidants that may boost your metabolism and increase fat burning .

This same effect also applies to matcha, a highly concentrated type of powdered green tea that contains the same beneficial ingredients as regular green tea.

2. Puerh Tea

Also known as pu'er or pu-erh tea, puerh tea is a type of Chinese black tea that has been fermented.

It is often enjoyed after a meal, and has an earthy aroma that tends to develop the longer it's stored.

Some animal studies have shown that puerh tea may lower blood sugar and blood triglycerides. And studies in animals and humans have shown that puerh tea may be able to help enhance weight loss.

In one study, 70 men were given either a capsule of puerh tea extract or a placebo. After three months, those taking the puerh tea capsule lost approximately 2.2 pounds (1 kg) more than the placebo group.

Another study in rats had similar findings, showing that puerh tea extract had an anti-obesity effect and helped suppress weight gain .

Current research is limited to puerh tea extract, so more research is needed to see if the same effects apply to drinking it as a tea.

3. Black Tea

Black tea is a type of tea that has undergone more oxidation than other types, such as green, white or oolong teas.

Oxidation is a chemical reaction that happens when the tea leaves are exposed to the air, resulting in browning that causes the characteristic dark color of black tea.

There are many different types and blends of black tea available, including popular varieties like Earl Grey and English breakfast.

Several studies have found that black tea could be effective when it comes to weight control.

One study of 111 people found that drinking three cups of black tea each day for three months significantly increased weight loss and reduced waist circumference, compared to drinking a caffeine-matched control beverage.

Some theorize that black tea's potential weight loss effects may be because it's high in flavones, a type of plant pigment with antioxidant properties.

A study followed 4,280 adults over 14 years. It found that those with a higher flavone intake from foods and beverages like black tea had a lower body mass index (BMI) than those with a lower flavone intake.

However, this study looks only at the association between BMI and flavone intake. Further research is needed to account for other factors that may be involved.

4. Oolong Tea

Oolong tea is a traditional Chinese tea that has been partially oxidized, putting it somewhere between green tea and black tea in terms of oxidation and color.

It is often described as having a fruity, fragrant aroma and a unique flavor, though these can vary significantly depending on the level of oxidation.

Several studies have shown that oolong tea could help enhance weight loss by improving fat burning and speeding up metabolism.

In one study, 102 overweight or obese people drank oolong tea every day for six weeks, which may have helped reduce both their body weight and body fat. The researchers proposed the tea did this by improving the metabolism of fat in the body .

Another small study gave men either water or tea for a three-day period, measuring their metabolic rates. Compared to water, oolong tea increased energy expenditure by 2.9%, the equivalent of burning an additional 281 calories per day, on average .

While more studies on the effects of oolong tea are needed, these findings show that oolong could be potentially beneficial for weight loss.

5. White Tea

White tea stands out among other types of tea because it is minimally processed and harvested while the tea plant is still young.

White tea has a distinct flavor very different from other types of tea. It tastes subtle, delicate and slightly sweet.

The benefits of white tea are well-studied, and range from improving oral health to killing cancer cells in some test-tube studies.

Though further research is needed, white tea could also help when it comes to losing weight and body fat.

Studies show that white tea and green tea have comparable amounts of catechins, which may help enhance weight loss .

Furthermore, one test-tube study showed that white tea extract increased the breakdown of fat cells while preventing the formation of new ones .

However, keep in mind that this was a test-tube study, so it's unclear how the effects of white tea may apply to humans.

Additional studies are needed to confirm the potential beneficial effects of white tea when it comes to fat loss.

6. Herbal Tea

Herbal teas involve the infusion of herbs, spices and fruits in hot water.

They differ from traditional teas because they do not typically contain caffeine, and are not made from the leaves of Camellia sinensis.

Popular herbal tea varieties include rooibos tea, ginger tea, rosehip tea and hibiscus tea.

Although the ingredients and formulations of herbal teas can vary significantly, some studies have found that herbal teas may help with weight reduction and fat loss.

In one animal study, researchers gave obese rats an herbal tea, and found that it reduced body weight and helped normalize hormone levels.

Rooibos tea is a type of herbal tea that may be especially effective when it comes to fat burning.

One test-tube study showed that rooibos tea increased fat metabolism and helped block the formation of fat cells.

However, further studies in humans are needed to look into the effects of herbal teas like rooibos on weight loss

Though many people drink tea solely for its soothing quality and delicious taste, each cup may also pack many health benefits.

Replacing high-calorie beverages like juice or soda with tea could help reduce overall calorie intake and lead to weight loss.

Some animal and test-tube studies have also shown that certain types of tea may help increase weight loss while blocking fat cell formation.

However, studies in humans are needed to investigate this further.

Additionally, many types of tea are especially high in beneficial compounds like flavones and catechins, which could aid in weight loss as well.

Coupled with a healthy diet and regular exercise, a cup or two of tea each day could help you boost weight loss and prevent harmful belly fat

How many times you have to do intermittent fasting

Now that you understand how to implement an intermittent fasting schedule, it raises a question: How often should you fast?

The answer varies from individual to individual. Most individuals implement the above schedules every week or every other week. If you're new to fasting, start with a moderate schedule, trying it every other week or every three weeks. If your body adapts well, aim for a regular, weekly schedule.

There's no wrong answer here. Pay close attention to how your body responds to your fasting schedule, and adjust as needed. Keep in mind that life changes can happen. You may need to tweak your schedule to allow for social gatherings, vacations and physical activity or competition.

In general, once or twice a week is an optimal frequency to perform intermittent fasting.

What not to eat during intermittent fasting

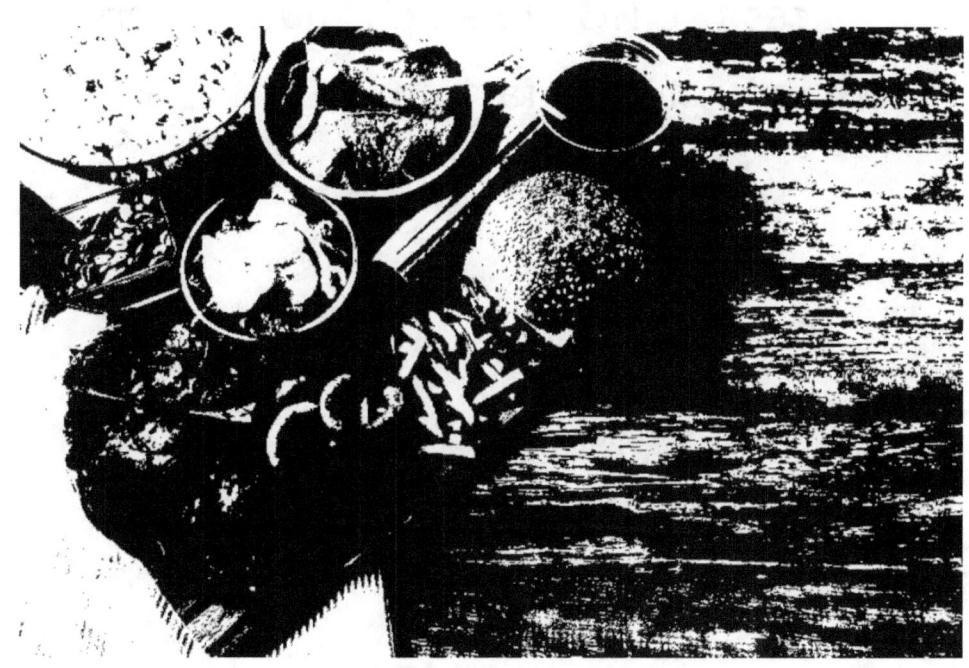

Any source of calories should be avoided during the period of intermittent fasting. So also all the oils and obviously sugars.

Any solid food should be avoided, including fruits, seeds and vegetables. Even shredded versions, extracts and juices are NOT used during the period of intermittent fasting.

Who should not do intermittent fasting

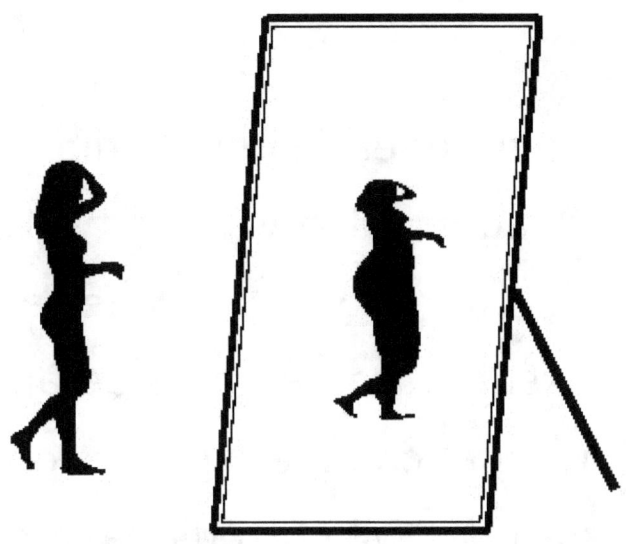

If you suffer or have suffered from eating disorders, it is not recommended to face any type of calorie restriction.

It is not appropriate for children to follow an intermittent fast.

Women in general should address it in the less aggressive version by 16 hours no more than 1-2 times a week. In fact, some women may be affected by hormonal changes (increased testosterone) which could lead to amenorrhea.

If the woman suffers from infertility she should avoid intermittent fasting.

In any case of pre-existing conditions it is necessary to discuss with your doctor to see if in the specific case it is advantageous to deal with the practice of intermittent fasting.

Who can deal with intermittent fasting

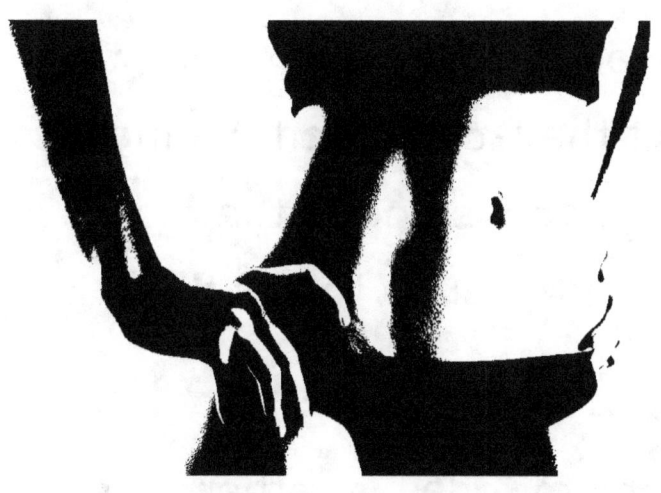

In general, boys are the ones who only benefit from intermittent fasting.All people (except children) are healthy, especially if overweight can benefit enormously from intermittent fasting.

As indicated in the initial part of the article, the human being in the course of its evolution has always had to confront the lack of food. Eating less and less often is one of the most natural and healthy things there is.

The problem today is rather in the sense of excess. How many diseases are caused by unhealthy foods consumed in excess!

Intermittent fasting is the (simple)
turn we need

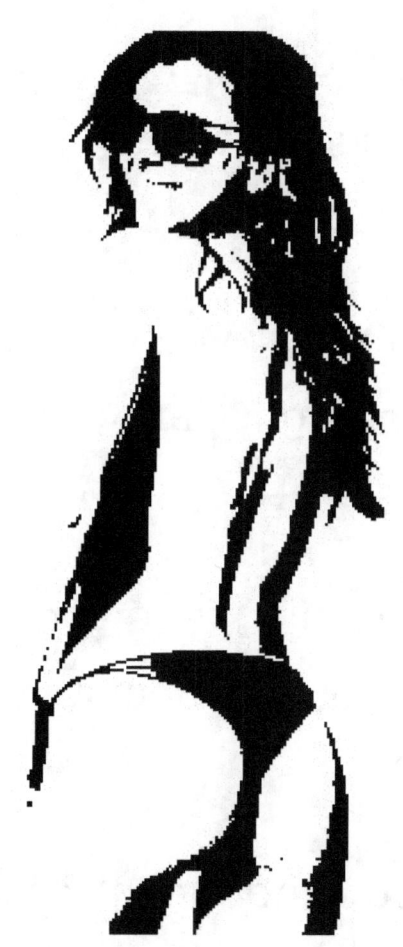

... It is appropriate to correct this
trend as soon as possible by turning

to the healthy habit of intermittently fasting.

There is a way of saying oriental wisdom that suggests ...

"No matter how far you've gotten away from the right path ... turn!"

The important thing is to correct yourself and do it immediately.

The more you continue in the same (wrong) direction under the influence of inertia, the more you will drift away: turning, now!

Conclusions

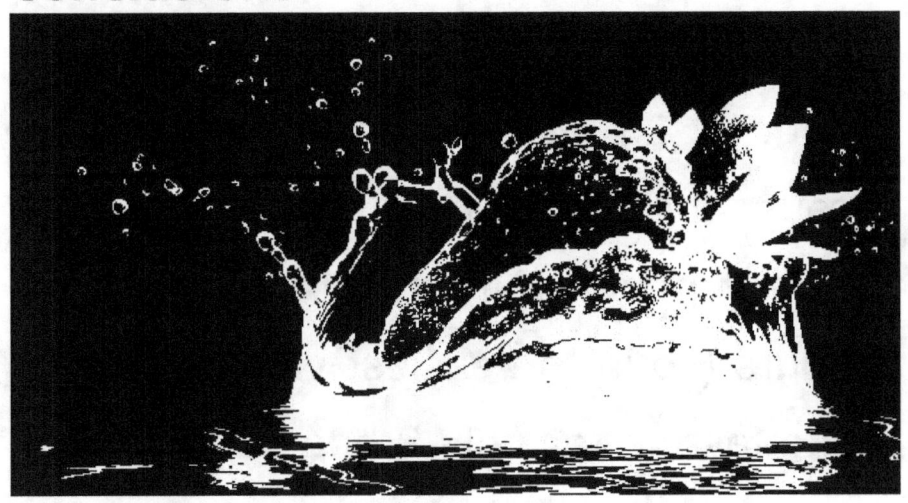

Are you lazy but want to do something more to regain health and fitness?

Intermittent fasting has all the characteristics to unleash a great therapeutic, protective and slimming power.

There is nothing healthier, simpler and cheaper than to stop eating for 16-24 hours 1-2 times a week. You can also count the 7-8 hours of sleep in the total number of intermittent fasting hours (so in the easiest version it is like fasting for only 8 hours!).

On the practical side, fasting intermittently also facilitates life. In fact, skipping a couple of meals every now and then eliminates the need to prepare them and you recover some time to devote to something else.

Motivation: Intermittet fasting success stories

Intermittent Fasting Success Stories

1. lucy's Story

After one year of 4:3 intermittent fasting, I've lost 39.8kg (6 stone 3.8lb). My body mass index (BMI) has reduced by 12.28, down to 36.79 from 49.07. I have had to throw many of my old clothes out because they have become loose and comical.

During the second half of my fasting (the latter six months of the twelve), I experienced long plateau periods, meaning little weight loss was apparent due to my metabolism slowing and my body burning fewer calories, strangely, these plateaus seem to only occur when approaching a weight-loss milestone (130kgs, 120kgs), and were usually followed by an abrupt and substantial loss of weight. Whilst I am aware that plateau is quite common around the six to nine-month mark of dieting, I am hoping to get past it and speed up my weight loss process.

I find it is easy to do after a year. On most fasting days, I often eat nothing at all, and sometimes continue the fasting until my afternoon meal the next day if I am not overly hungry.

All in all, I feel fantastic, although I still carry a lot of body weight, I feel much lighter on my feet and more energetic than I was before. I also feel as though my strength and endurance have improved.

2. Tabatha's Story

I have had to throw all of my old clothes out and purchase an entirely new wardrobe since fasting. I have just turned 65, my weight is now 127lbs, my body-fat ratio is 27.3%, I have a BMI of 20.2%, and a 29-inch waistline. I am feeling very good and am planning on continuing my dietary plan for a few years or more, to ensure I remain healthy and enjoy the years I have left to the fullest.Here's how I achieved it:

I use the 5:2 method, whereby I only had to count calories on two days out of seven in a week.During the early stages of the regime I would nibble on snacks the evening before fast days to load up on calories, and the next day whilst fasting I would be thinking about food non-stop. However, this didn't last that long, and it wasn't long before I stopped snacking even on non-fasting days.

I found that distributing my calorie intake between the times of 12 pm and 7 pm, and skipping breakfast everyday (as I had always struggled to consume and enjoy breakfast consistently) worked wonders for me.

Once I hit my target weight in March, I decided to change to a 6:1 plan to see how my body would react. What I found was that even when I didn't fast at all throughout the week by adhering to the 7-hour window (between 12 pm and 7 pm), I was still steadily losing weight. After reading some intermittent fasting success stories, I found that this seven-hour window had been useful for others, too.

After going on holiday, I put on a few pounds, but once I had returned home and re-established my seven hour eating window, I lost the extra holiday weight within two weeks.

3. Jina's Story

After deciding that it was time to change my eating habits and attain what is considered a healthy weight for my age, I decided to try 5:2 intermittent fasting. I began fasting on the 1st of July 2013, and my body weight was 170lbs (12st 2lbs), as of today (September 24th, 2013), my body weight has dropped to 145lbs (10st 5lbs).

I generally fast on Mondays, Thursdays, or Fridays, depending on impending commitments. I fast from evening meal to evening meal, for 24 hour periods. At one point I attempted to fast for a 36-hour period, but this caused me to have trouble sleeping and left my stomach feeling extremely empty. For this reason, I continued to consume a small, nutritious meal in the evening on fast days.

I began diet by eating complex carbohydrates (whole meal bread, spaghetti, and brown rice), but have swapped these starchy foods for courgette "spaghetti" and cauliflower "rice", which are delicious alternatives. I have abstained from eating all white carbohydrates, and I log everything I eat into an app on my smart phone which records the calorie content. This provides me with helpful statistics and ensures I adhere to my weight loss goals.

Since fasting I have gone from a size 16 to a size 10, and I am feeling very positive about my appearance. I have read many intermittent fasting success stories to ascertain that I am not alone in my success. I will continue to maintain my fasting plan and work toward my target weight of 139lbs (9st 13lbs).

4. Maria's Story

After putting a few stone on during menopause, I decided to try intermittent fasting to lose my post-menopausal weight. Starting in September/October time in 2012, I first implemented the 5:2 diet plan but soon began a 16/8 method, wherein I would have 16 hour fast periods and 8 hour eating windows every day. I get great displeasure from counting calories so I found this method best suited for more – simply skip breakfast and don't nibble in the evenings, how hard could it be? Since fasting I have gone from 140lbs (10st) to around 112/117lbs (8st to 8st 4lbs).

At first I would eat whatever I wanted during the 8 hour eating period of each day, with little to no concern of healthy/nutritious meals. Before long, I began to implement healthier meals and really noticed the benefits from doing so.

At first, weight loss was slow, which can be disheartening, but I persevered and eventually lost the weight I wanted to. I feel brilliant, full of energy and life, and my friends and family say I look better than I have for many years. Intermittent fasting truly has changed my life for the better. I would definitely recommend this method of eating, and this way of life to anyone.

ITERMITTENT FASTING STARTER COOKBOOK

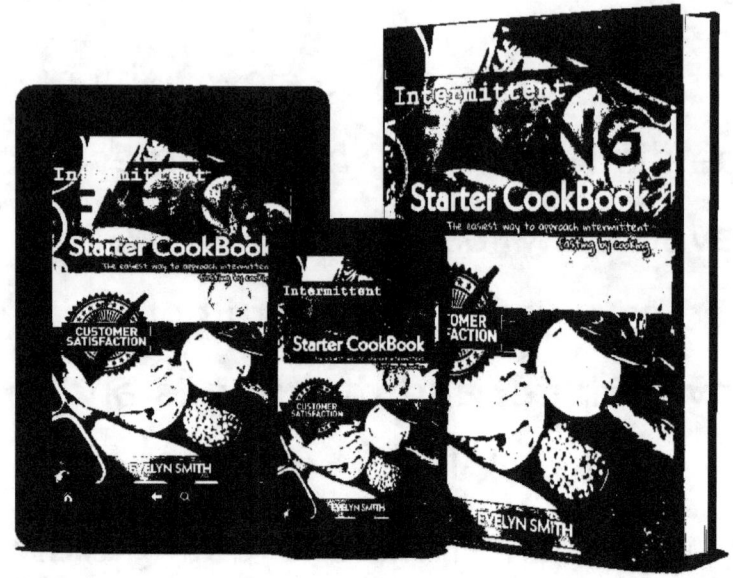

INTRODUCTION

Modern society has an obsession with food and with eating. Everywhere you turn, there are advertisements for different food products and food just seems to be constantly pushed at us.

At the same time, food can have a strong impact on our emotions and many of the products in our stores are made and marketed in a way that makes us crave them.

Our obsession with food is incredibly unhealthy and dangerous – but how do we break out of that? After all, we do still need to eat to live.

One interesting idea is that perhaps our eating patterns are wrong. Do we really need to eat three meals (plus snacks) every day? Is being hungry actually something we should be avoiding at all costs? Or, might it be, that hunger is much more important than we typically assume?

Those concepts are why there has been increased interest and research into a biological process called autophagy, along with the implications that an autophagy diet might have for our health and weight.

Intermittent Fasting and Keto: How Are They Related?

The topics of ketosis and intermittent fasting often fall within the same conversation. Why? Because intermittent fasting can be used as a tool to reach ketosis.

When you fast, you deplete your body of glycogen stores. Once glycogen stores are gone, fat stores are released into your bloodstream to be converted into energy molecules (ketones) in the liver.

This is the metabolic process we call ketosis.

Just as intense and prolonged exercise (particularly HIIT training or lifting weights) can help induce a ketogenic state, intermittent fasting will make you enter ketosis faster than following a keto diet alone.

There are many more overlaps between intermittent fasting and keto, which you'll learn about below.

What Is Ketosis?

Ketosis is the process of burning ketone bodies for energy.

On a regular carb-based diet, your body burns glucose, not ketones, as its primary fuel source. Excess glucose is stored as glycogen. When your body is deprived of glucose (due to exercise, intermittent fasting or a ketogenic diet) it will turn to glycogen for energy. Only after glycogen is depleted will your body start burning fat.

A ketogenic diet, which is a low carb, high fat diet, creates a metabolic shift that allows your body to break down fat into ketone bodies in the liver for energy. There are three main ketone bodies found in your blood, urine, and breath:

Acetoacetate: It's the ketone that's created first. It can either be converted into beta-hydroxybutyrate or turned into acetone.

Acetone: Created spontaneously from the breakdown of acetoacetate. It's the most volatile ketone and is often detectable on the breath when someone first goes into ketosis.

Beta-hydroxybutyrate (BHB): This is the ketone that's actually used for energy and the most abundant in your blood once you're fully into ketosis. It's the type that's found in exogenous ketones and what blood tests measure.

Now, how does intermittent fasting fit into ketosis?

What Is Intermittent Fasting and How Does It Relate to Ketosis?

Intermittent fasting consists of eating within a specific feeding window and not eating the remaining hours of the day. Every person, whether they're aware of it or not, fasts overnight from dinner to breakfast, for example.

There are many approaches to intermittent fasting — some people fast for 16-20 hours periods, on alternate days or following a 24-hour day fast.

If you want to start fasting, one popular version is the 16/8 method, where you eat within an 8-hour eating window (ex. 11:00 a.m. to 7:00 p.m.), followed by a 16-hour fasting window.

Other fasting schedules include the 20/4 or 14/10 methods. Others practice 24-hour fasts once or twice per week.

Intermittent fasting can put you in ketosis faster because your cells will quickly consume your glycogen stores and start burning fat for fuel.

But what about after you get into ketosis? Is intermittent fasting worth doing consistently?

Short answer: Yes. Here's why it can be a great addition to your health toolbox:

Ketosis vs. Intermittent Fasting: Physical Benefits

Both the keto diet and intermittent fasting are effective tools for:

Healthy weight-loss

Fat loss — not muscle loss

Balancing cholesterol levels

Improving insulin sensitivity

Keeping blood sugar levels stable

KETO FOR WEIGHT LOSS, FAT LOSS AND IMPROVED CHOLESTEROL

The ketogenic diet drastically decreases your carb intake, forcing your body to burn fat rather than glucose, making it an effective tool for weight loss.

While individual results vary, keto has consistently led to a reduction in weight and body fat percentage in a wide range of situations.

In a 2017 study, subjects who followed a low carbohydrate keto meal plan significantly decreased body weight, body fat percentage and fat mass, losing an average of 7.6 pounds and 2.6% body fat while maintaining lean muscle mass.

Similarly, a 2004 study observing the long-term effects of a ketogenic diet in obese patients found that weight and body mass of the patients decreased dramatically over the course of two years. Those who drastically reduced their carbohydrate intake saw a significant decrease in LDL (bad) cholesterol, triglycerides and improved insulin sensitivity.

In 2012, a study compared a ketogenic diet to eating fewer calories in obese children and adults. The results showed children following the keto diet lost significantly more body weight, fat mass and total waist circumference. They also showed a dramatic decrease in insulin levels, a biomarker of Type 2 diabetes

INTERMITTENT FASTING FOR FAT LOSS AND MAINTAINING MUSCLE MASS

Research has shown intermittent fasting can be an efficient weight loss tool and sometimes more effective than simply cutting calories.

In one study, intermittent fasting was shown to be as effective as continuous calorie restriction in fighting obesity[*]. In studies done by the NIH, there was reported weight loss with over 84% of participants — no matter which fasting schedule they chose[*].

Like ketosis, intermittent fasting increases fat loss while maintaining lean muscle mass. In one study, researchers concluded that fasting resulted in greater weight loss (while preserving muscle) than a low-calorie diet, even though the total caloric intake was the same[*].

The bottom line is, if you're trying to lose fat, doing ketosis and IF can be a huge help. But that's not where the benefits stop.

Ketosis vs. Intermittent Fasting: Mental Benefits

Beyond their physiological benefits, both intermittent fasting and ketosis provide various mental benefits. Both have been scientifically shown to:

Boost memory

Improve mental clarity and focus

Prevent neurological diseases including Alzheimer's and epilepsy

KETO FOR IMPROVING BRAIN FOG AND MEMORY

On a carb-based diet, the fluctuations in your blood sugar levels can cause fluctuations in energy levels (known as as sugar highs and sugar crashes).

In ketosis, your brain uses a more consistent source of fuel: ketones from your fat stores, resulting in better productivity and mental performance.

Why? Because your brain is the most energy-consuming organ in your body. When you have a clean and consistent energy supply from ketones, your brain functions better.

On top of that, ketones are better at protecting your brain.Studies show ketone bodies may have antioxidant properties that protect your brain cells from free radicals, oxidative stress and damage[*].

In one study performed on adults with impaired memory, the rise of BHB ketones in their blood helped improve cognition[*].

If you have a hard time staying focused, your neurotransmitters may be to blame. Your brain has two main neurotransmitters: glutamate and GABA.

Glutamate helps you form new memories, learn complicated concepts and gets your brain cells to communicate with each other. Any time you text, talk or think, you can thank glutamate for helping.

GABA is what helps control glutamate. Glutamate can make your brain cells overly excited. If this happens too often, it can cause brain cells to stop working and eventually die. GABA is there to control and slow down glutamate[*]. When GABA levels are low, glutamate reigns free and you experience mental fog.

What does this have to do with ketones? Ketones prevent damage to brain cells by processing excess glutamate into GABA. Since ketones increase GABA and decrease glutamate, they aid in preventing cell damage, avoiding cell death and improving your mental focus.

In other words, ketones help keep your GABA and glutamate levels balanced so your brain stays sharp.

INTERMITTENT FASTING EFFECTS ON STRESS LEVELS AND COGNITIVE FUNCTION

Fasting has been shown improve your memory, reduce oxidative stress, and preserve your learning capabilities[*].

Scientists believe this happens because IF forces your cells to perform better. Because your cells are under mild stress while fasting, the best cells adapt to this stress by enhancing their own ability to cope, while the weakest cells die.

This is similar to the stress your body undergoes when you hit the gym. Exercise is a form of stress your body endures to improve and get stronger, as long as you rest enough after your workouts. This also applies for intermittent fasting: As long as you continue to alternate between regular eating habits and fasting, it will continue to benefit you.

All of this means both ketosis and IF can help improve your cognitive function thanks to the protective and energizing effects of ketones, as well as the mild cellular stress caused by fasting.

The Perks Of Fasting And Doing Keto

The ketogenic diet and intermittent fasting have many of the same health benefits. Why? Because both methods can have the same result: a metabolic state known as ketosis.

Ketosis has many physical and mental benefits, from weight and fat loss to improved stress levels, brain function, and longevity.

Does intermittent fasting always cause ketosis? Absolutely not. If you take a more mild approach to intermittent fasting (for example, eating within an 8-hour window), you probably won't enter ketosis (especially if you eat a high amount of carbs during that window).

Plus, not everyone who tries intermittent fasting aims to enter ketosis. If someone who fasts also eats high-carb foods, there is a very good chance they'll never enter ketosis.

If, on the other hand, ketosis is the goal, ketoers can use intermittent fasting as a tool to get there and improve their overall health.

INTERMITTENT FASTING RECIPES: Low-Carb & Keto California AVO Omelet

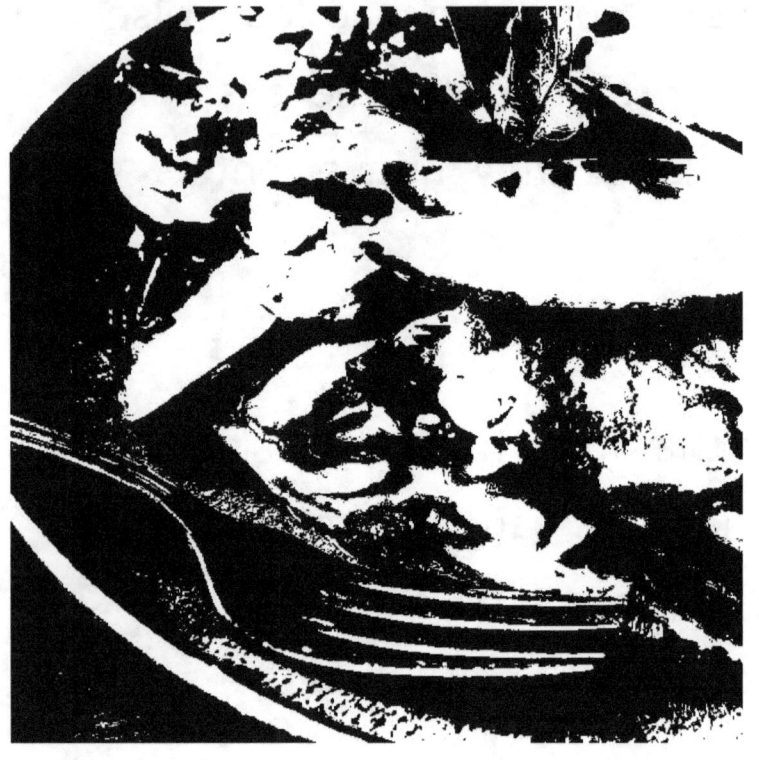

This keto omelet is a great low-carb, high-fat breakfast option that's packed with flavor, healthy fats, protein and electrolytes from shrimp, avocado, red bell peppers, green onions, and plenty of butter — what's an omelet without butter? If you are dairy-free, simply swap for duck fat or olive oil.

This keto recipe yields one very large omelet or two small omelets. Feel free to make this quick and serve by cutting in half or if you're the one meal a day (OMAD) style keto eater who practices intermittent fasting, this makes a great large meal! Serve it up with extra hot sauce on the side for a fiery kick!

Save on Prep Time and Cook Your Bacon in Advance

This recipe uses crispy bacon — always keep some cooked bacon in the fridge so you can use it in meals and save on prep time.

There are two ways to cook bacon. Crisping up bacon in a skillet is ideal for cooking just a few slices, while baking in the oven is better for large batches.

How to Cook Bacon in a Skillet?

Place the slices in a hot skillet. Add about 1/2 cup (120 ml) water and cook on medium until the water evaporates and the bacon is crisped up, for 10-15 minutes. As the fat renders, the bacon will cook and crisp up in it. Use a slotted spoon to transfer the crisped up bacon to a plate, leaving the rendered fat in the skillet.

If you're using leaner bacon slices, you can lightly grease the skillet with ghee, lard or duck fat and then cook for 2-3 minutes per side until crisp. You can then store your bacon in the fridge for up to four days or freeze for up to three months.

How to Cook Bacon in the Oven?

To cook bacon in the oven, preheat the oven to 190 °C/ 375 °F (fan assisted), or 210 °C/ 410 °F (conventional). Line a baking tray with baking paper. Lay the bacon strips out flat on the baking paper, leaving space so they don't overlap. Place the tray in the oven and cook for about 10-15 minutes until golden brown. The time depends on the thickness of the bacon slices. When done, remove from the oven and set aside to cool down.

If you have time, use lower temperature setting and cook your bacon at 160 °C/ 320 °F (fan assisted), or 180 °C/ 355 °F (conventional) for 25-30 minutes. The bacon cooks more evenly and it's less likely to burn it.

Ingredients (makes 2 servings)

6 large eggs, whisked

1/4 tsp lemon juice

1/4 tsp hot sauce (you can make your own Sriracha Sauce)

1/4 tsp sea salt

3 tbsp butter, ghee or duck fat (43 g/ 1.5 oz)

10-12 pieces cooked shrimp, peeled and deveined (115 g/ 4 oz)

2 tbsp minced parsley or cilantro

1/4 cup minced red bell pepper (37 g/ 1.3 oz)

1 medium green onion, sliced (15 g/ 0.5 oz)

1 large avocado, sliced (200 g/ 7.1 oz)

2 slices cooked bacon (32 g/ 1.1 oz)

Instructions

1) In a small bowl whisk the eggs, lemon juice, hot sauce, and salt together. You can make one large omelet and eat half per serving, or make 2 regular omelets.

2) Heat the butter in a large nonstick pan over medium-low heat. Once melted pour in the whisked eggs. Cook lifting the edges with a spatula and tilting the pan to allow uncooked egg to run under the omelet until set but still moist on top. If you're making 2 smaller omelets, cook them in batches.

3) Arrange the shrimp, parsley, bell pepper, green onion, avocado and bacon across the top of the omelet. Gently fold in half and cook another 2-3 minutes until cooked through.

4) Serve immediately.

Ingredient nutritional breakdown (per serving)

	Net carbs	Protein	Fat	Calories	
Eggs, free-range or organic	1,1g	18,8g	14,3	215kcal	
Lemon juice, fresh	0g	0g	og	okcal	
Sriracha Hot Chili Sauce, homemade	0,1g	0g	og	1kcal	
Salt, sea salt	0g	0g	0g	0kcal	
Butter, unsalted, grass-fed	0g	0,2g	17,3 g	153 kcal	
Prawns, shrimp	0,5g	11,6g	1g	60 kcal	
Parsley, fresh (spices)	0,1g	0,1g	0g	1 kcal	

Peppers, red bell, fresh	0,7g	0,2g	0,1g	6 kcal
Spring onion, scallion, green onion, fresh	0,4g	0,1g	0g	2 kcal
Avocado, fresh	1.8g	2g	14,7g	161 kcal
Bacon, crispy (bacon grease removed)	0g	2,4g	0,8 g	17 kcal
Total per serving	4,7g	35,4	48,2	615 kcal

Keto Buffalo Chicken Chopped Salad

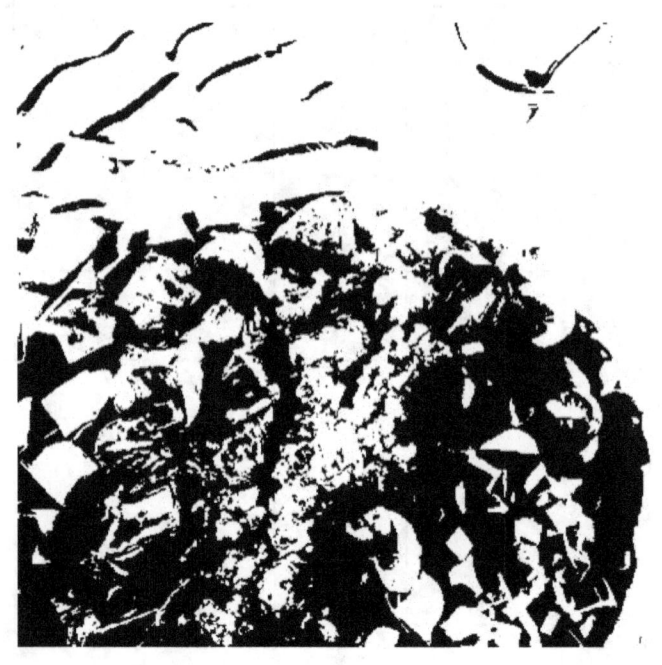

This chopped Buffalo chicken blue cheese salad bowl is one of my favorite low-carb salads! I love the crunch of all of the fresh veggies (those carrots!) plus the tangy buffalo chicken and creamy avocado.

Really, with bacon, blue cheese, and buffalo sauce how could you go wrong? This keto salad is great for meal prep as it also holds up really well (minus the avocado) in the refrigerator for a pre-made lunch option. Just be sure to cut the avocado fresh to prevent it from turning brown.

This recipe makes three regular servings or two large servings. A large serving (half of this recipe) is ideal for those who practice intermittent fasting and need a nutritious meal to break their fasting window.

How many carbs are in chili sauce?

Watch out for added sugars in condiments such as chili/hot sauce. Most of these products are not correctly labeled. For example, Frank's RedHot Sauce lists values "per tablespoon" which are rounded down to zero, resulting in seemingly zero-carb values per any amounts. That's also one of the reasons branded products are not reliable when it comes to food tracking.

While added sugar is not always an issue (contrary to common beliefs), eating too many hidden carbs could be what's stalling your progress.

If you want to be absolutely sure and have a complete control over your carb intake, you can always make your own condiments, including Sriracha Chili Sauce and Ranch Dressing. They are easy to make and taste amazing — much better than most store-bought products!

Hands-on 10 minutes Overall 20-25 minutes

Ingredients (makes 3 servings)
Buffalo chicken:
285 g cooked diced chicken (10 oz)
3 tbsp butter, melted (43 g/ 1.5 oz)
1/4 cup Frank's RedHot sauce or Sriracha chili sauce (60 ml/ 2 fl oz) - you can make your own chili sauce
Salad:
1 large romaine lettuce, chopped (285 g/ 10 oz)
4 slices crisped up bacon, crumbled (64 g/ 2.3 oz)

1 small carrot, diced (60 g/ 2.1 oz)

1/4 cup banana peppers or green bell peppers (30 g/ 1.1 oz)

4 green onions, thinly sliced (60 g/ 2.1 oz)

1/2 cup halved cherry tomatoes (75 g/ 2.6 oz)

1/4 cup crumbled blue cheese (34 g/ 1.2 oz)

1 large avocado, diced (200 g/ 7.1 oz)

Dressing:

6 tbsp ranch dressing (90 ml/ 3.2 fl oz) - you can make your own Keto Ranch Dressing

2 tbsp crumbled blue cheese (20 g/ 0.7 oz)

1 tbsp buffalo sauce or Sriracha chili sauce (15 ml)

Instructions

1) In a medium bowl toss the chicken with the melted butter and buffalo sauce.

2) In a small jar mix together the dressing ingredients.

3) Divide the salad fillings between three salad bowls, top with chicken and drizzle with dressing.

4) Serve immediately or store in the fridge for up to 2 days.

Ingredient nutritional breakdown (per serving)

	Net carb	Protein	Fat	Calories
Chicken breast, cooked, boiled	0 g	27,5 g	2,9 g	143 ckal
Butter, unsalted, grass-fed	0g	0,1 g	11,5 g	102 Kcal
Sriracha Hot Chili Sauce, homemade (KetoDiet blog)	1,8 g	0,5 g	1,2 g	20 kcal
Lettuce, Romaine	1,1 g	1,2 g	O,3 g	16 kcal
Bacon, crispy	0 g	6,4 g	2,1 g	45 ckal

(bacon grease removed)				
Carrot, fresh	1,4 g	0,2 g	O g	8 kcal
Banana Peppers (Giant)	0,2 g	0 g	0 g	1 Kcal
Spring onion, scallion, green onion, fresh	0,9 g	0,4 g	0 g	6 kcal
Tomatoes, cherry, fresh, all varieties	0,5 g	0,2 g	0,1 g	4 kcal
Cheese, blue	0,3 g	2,4 g	3,2 g	40 kcal
Avocado, fresh	1,2 g	1,3 g	9,8 g	107 kcal
Keto Ranch Dressing	0,7 g	0,5 g	13 g	121 kcal

Cheese, blue	0,2 g	1,4 g	1,9 g	24 kcal
Sriracha Hot Chili Sauce, homemade	0,5 g	0,1 g	0,3 g	5 ckal
Total per serving	8,7 g	42,2 g	46,4 g	642 kcal

Low-Carb Steak Taco Bowl

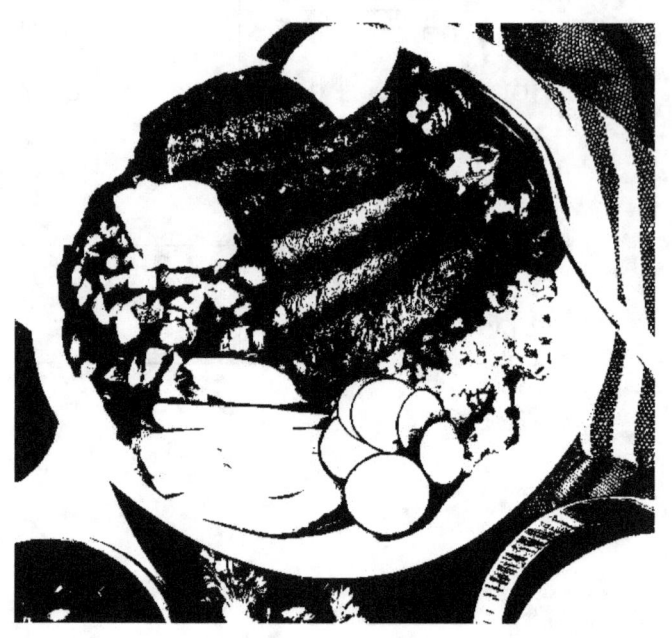

This low-carb Steak Taco Bowl is an easy meal and a great lunchbox option that can be ready in less than 20 minutes. Even less if you prep the bowl while the steak is searing and resting, or if you use leftover steak from last night's dinner.

It's packed with flavor using simple fresh ingredients: cilantro lime cauliflower rice, juicy steak, avocado, sour cream, homemade tomato salsa, crunchy jalapeños, and radishes. Yum! This recipe can easily be scaled up to make multiple servings as well.

Tip: This easy taco bowl is a great option for those who practice intermittent fasting as just one serving will provide enough protein, fat and electrolytes to keep you full and nourished for longer.

Hands-on 10 minutes Overall 20 minutes

Ingredients (makes 1 serving)

Steak Bowl:
1 small filet steak or any of your favorite steaks (150 g/ 5.3 oz)
1 tbsp butter or ghee (15 ml)
salt and pepper, to taste
1 cup cauliflower rice, cooked (120 g/ 4.2 oz)
2 tbsp minced cilantro
1 tsp lime juice

Toppings:

1/2 medium avocado, sliced (75 g/ 2.7 oz)

1/4 cup Simple Tomato Salsa or our Radish Salsa or Summer Vegetable Salsa (50 g/ 1.8 oz)

1 tbsp sour cream (12 g/ 0.4 oz)

1/2 jalapeño pepper, sliced (7 g/ 0.3 oz)

2 radishes, thinly sliced (15 g/ 0.5 oz)

Optional: more cilantro and lime wedges for garnish

Instructions

1) Heat the butter over medium-high heat in a small skillet. Season the filet with salt and pepper. Sear the filet for 4 to 8 minutes per side, depending on how you want the steak cooked.

2) Transfer to a cutting board and allow to rest while you assemble the rest of the bowls.

3) In a bowl, mix the cooked cauliflower rice with cilantro and lime juice.

Note: You can cook the cauliflower rice by steaming,

microwaving, pan roasting or oven baking

4)Top with other toppings. Thinly slice the steak and place on top of the cauliflower rice.

5) Serve immediately or store in the fridge for up to a day.

	Net carb	Protein	Fat	Calories
Filet mignon,beef tenderloin ,raw	0 g	29.4 g	27.2 g	371 kcal
ghee	0 g	0 g	15 g	136 kcal
salt, sea salt	0 g	0 g	0 g	0 kcal
pepper	0 g	0 g	0 g	0 kcal
Cauliflower rice homemade	3.6 g	2.3 g	0.3 g	30 kcal
Coriander (cilantro), fresh	0.1 g	0.2 g	0 g	2 kcal
Lime juice, fresh	1 g	0.1 g	0 g	3 kcal
Avocado, fresh	1.4 g	1.5 g	11 g	120 kcal

Simple Tomato Salsa - Pico De Gallo	1.7 g	0.4	0.1 g	12 kcal
Cream, sour	0.6 g	0.6 g	0.3 g	24 kcal
Peppers, jalapeno, raw	0.3 g	0.3 g	0.1 g	2 kcal
Radishes, raw	0.3 g	0.1 g	0 g	2 kcal
Total per serving	8.8 g	34.3 g	56.1 g	702 kcal

Low-Carb Butter Braised Cabbage with Crispy Ham

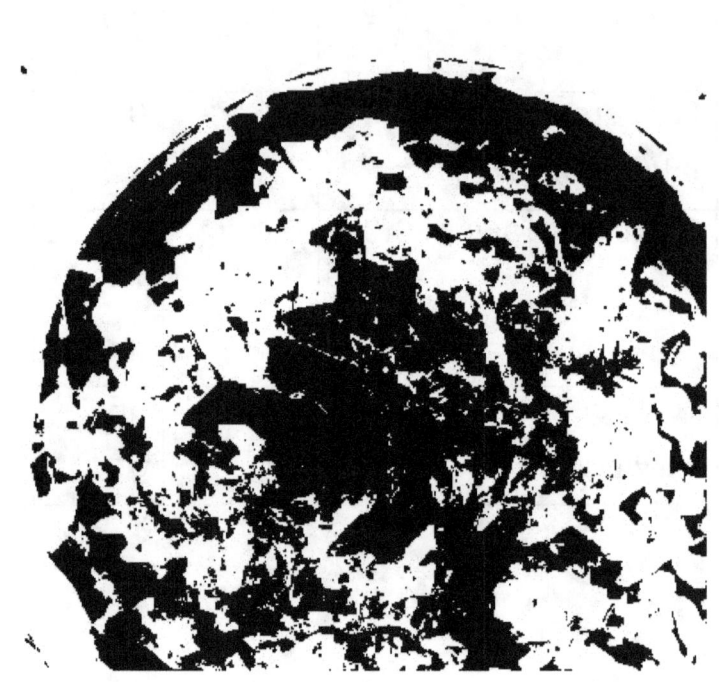

I was talking food and recipes with my foodie sister recently and she mentioned that her kids are weird, in that they love her butter braised cabbage.

I heard butter and I heard cabbage and my mind went, hmmmmm... Here is the result, soft, velvety cabbage in a rich buttery sauce.

This high-fat dish is ideal as a side with lean meat cuts such as pork tenderloin, beef sirloin, chicken breasts or white fish. If you practice intermittent fasting and only eat one or two high energy meals per day, feel free to serve it with fatty meat cuts such as pork belly, beef ribeye or fatty fish such as salmon.

I'm with her kids, I love it too! Enjoy!

Hands-on 10 minutes Overall 2 hours 15 minutes

Ingredients (makes 4 servings)

1/2 head white or green cabbage (600 g/ 1.3 lb)

2 sticks unsalted butter (225 g/ 8 oz)

sea salt, to taste

black pepper, to taste

6 slices prosciutto di Parma (90 g/ 3.2 oz)

Instructions

1) Slice cabbage and place it in a dutch oven or large saucepan.
2) Chop butter into chunks and sit on top of cabbage.
3) Put lid on pot and cook on low for about 2 hours, stirring every 15-20 minutes to prevent burning. Do not put water in.
4) Heat oven to 180 °C/ 355 °F (fan assisted), or 200 °C/ 400 °F (conventional). Place prosciutto on a rack over an

oven tray and cook for 10-15
minutes until crispy.

5) Cool, then crumble roughly into
a container.

6) Once cabbage is finished, serve
with a healthy grind of black
pepper and crumbled prosciutto
on top.

7) Store in a container in the
refrigerator for up to 4 days.

Total Carbs	8.7 grams
Fiber	3.8 grams
Net Carbs	5 grams
Protein	8.2 grams

Fat 48.4 grams	
of which Saturated 29.3 grams	
Calories 489 kcal	
Magnesium 19 mg (5% RDA)	
Potassium 269 mg (13% EMR)	
Macronutrient ratio: Calories from carbs (4%), protein (7%), fat (89%)	

Low-Carb Cheese & Bacon Stuffed Meat Pies

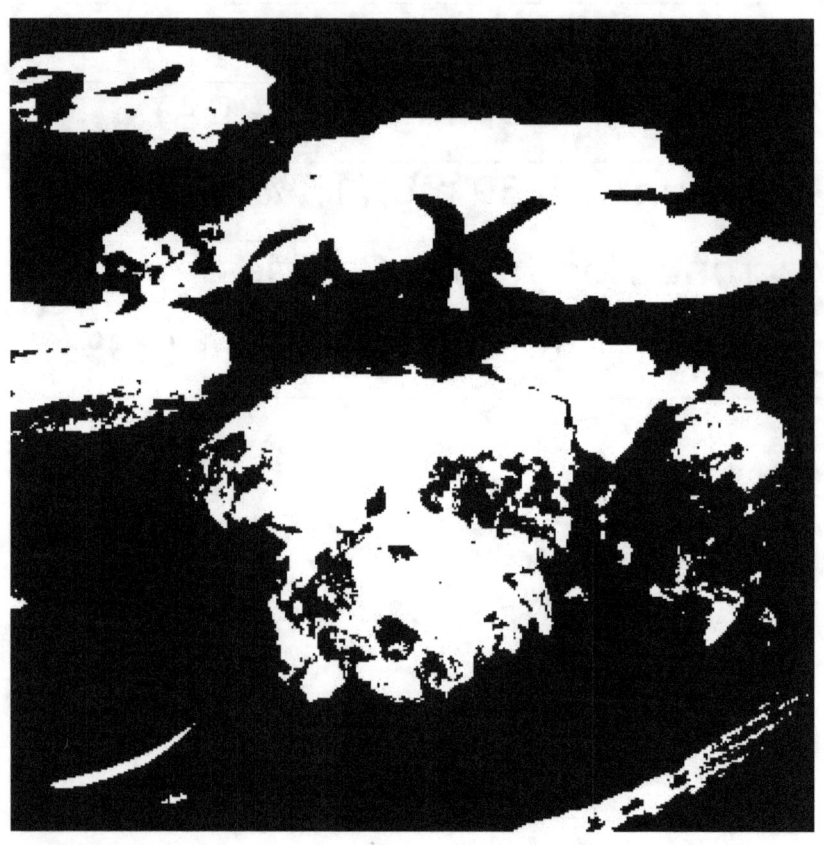

If there is anything that we love here in New Zeland , it's a meat pie with tomato sauce. Well, because I'm classy I used to love the beef, cheese and bacon pies and I'd be lying if I said that I haven't missed them.

These keto meat pies are satisfying enough to be served as a main dish with a side of dressed greens or on its own. It's a great option for those who practice intermittent fasting as it will provide enough fats and protein to break your fast.

I don't know how much I will get to enjoy these gluten-free meat pies though, as I have two hungry contractors in the house who have already requested them for their lunch tomorrow.

I'm guessing that they have missed pies too. Enjoy!

Hands-on 30 minutes Overall 1 hour 30 minutes

Ingredients (makes 6 mini meat pies)

Filling:

500 g ground beef (1.1 lb)

4 large slices bacon, chopped (120 g/ 4.2 oz)

1 small brown onion, chopped (g/ oz)

1 tbsp coconut aminos (15 ml)

2 tbsp tomato sauce/passata (30 ml)

1 cup beef stock or bone broth (240 ml/ 8 fl oz)

1/2 tsp xanthan gum

Pie crust:

2 1/4 cups shredded mozzarella cheese (250 g/ 8.8 oz)

1 cup + 2 tbsp shredded edam cheese (125 g/ 4.4 oz)

1/3 cup + 1 tbsp full-fat cream cheese (100 g/ 3.5 oz)

1 1/2 cups almond flour (150 g/ 5.3 oz)

2 large eggs

1 tsp onion powder

6 small chunks of sharp cheddar (66 g/ 2.3 oz)

Instructions

1) Cut the bacon into small strips and dice the onion.
2) Add to a skillet, along with the ground beef. Cook until just browned.
3) Add coconut aminos, passata, beef stock and xanthan gum and stir well to combine. Bring to the boil then reduce the heat and simmer for 30 minutes
4) Remove from the heat and let cool. Once mixture is cool, heat oven to 200 °C/ 400 °F (fan

assisted), or 220 °C/ 425 °F (conventional).

5) Prepare the pie crust. Place the cheeses and cream cheese into a large bowl and microwave for 1 minute. Remove and stir, then return for another 30 seconds. Repeat this once more. Add the almond meal, onion powder and eggs and mix well until you have a soft dough.

6) Divide into four parts and sit one portion aside. Cut each of the remaining three portions in half and then flatten them out into large circles (you will have a total of six circles).

7) Spray a six-hole oversized muffin pan and press the dough into each cup, making sure to leave overhang at the top as the dough will shrink while cooking. Bake for 10 minutes.

8) Remove and spoon some filling in to each cup. Press a chunk of cheddar into the centre.

9) Then top with the remaining filling.

10) Divide the reserved dough into six and flatten out into lids. Lay the lid on top of the pies and gently press around the edges to seal. Cut a couple of steam vents in top of each pie.

11) Return to the oven for 10-15 minutes until golden brown on top.

12) Eat warm, with sugar-free ketchup if you want to feel very Australian. If you can't find sugar-free, you can make your own keto ketchup in just a few minutes!

13) Store in the refrigerator for up to 5 days.

Ingredient nutritional breakdown (per meat pie)

Net carbs	Protein	Fat	Calories
Mozzarella cheese (low moisture, for pizza)			
2.3 g	9.9 g	8.2 g	123 kcal

Cheese, edam			
0.3 g 5.2 g 5.8 g 74 kcal			
Cream cheese, soft (full-fat)			
0.5 g 1.2 g 4.7 g 41 kcal			
Almond flour (blanched ground almonds, almond meal)			
2.2 g 5.4 g 13.1 g		148 kcal	
Eggs, free-range or organic			
0.1 g 2.1 g 1.6 g 24 kcal			
Onion powder, spices			
0.3 g 0 g	0 g	1 kcal	
Cheddar cheese			
0.3 g 2.5 g 3.7 g 44 kcal			
Beef, minced (ground), raw, grass-fed			
0 g	14.3 g	16.7 g	212 kcal
Bacon, streaky (high fat content), organic			

0 g	2.7 g	5 g	56 kcal

Onion, brown (yellow), raw

0.7 g	0.1 g	0 g	4 kcal

Coconut aminos (substitute to soy sauce)

0.2 g	0 g	0 g	1 kcal

Tomato sauce (passata), unsweetened

0.2 g	0.1 g	0 g	1 kcal

Beef bone broth

0.1 g	0.6 g	0.5 g	7 kcal

Xanthan gum, thickening agent

0 g	0 g	0 g	1 kcal

Total per meat pie

7.3 g	44.1 g	59.3 g	737 kcal

Salmon BLT Keto Sandwich

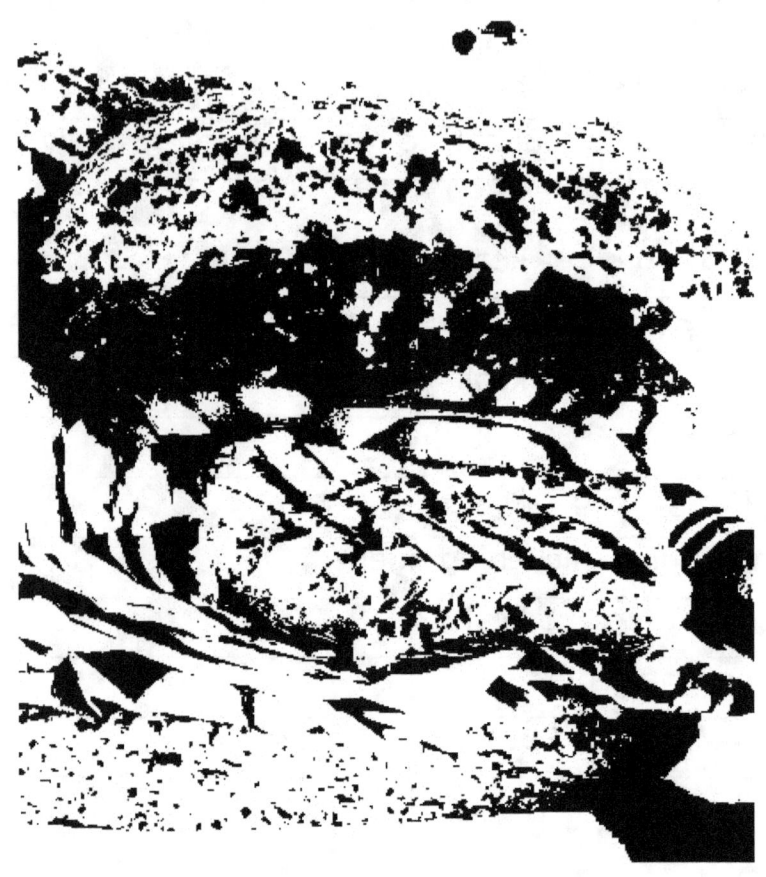

This keto Salmon BLT is an awesome low-carb and grain-free sandwich!

There's quite a few variations you could do as well:

Mix chipotles in adobo into the mayo

Add chile powder and lime juice to the mayo

Add fresh or roasted garlic to the mayo

Add sliced avocado to the sandwich

Add a slice of cheese such as cheddar, provolone or manchego

I could go on and on with a million different ideas, leave yours in the comments below!

We used the all-time favorite Keto Buns recipe for the bread here and they are perfect! I love keeping a batch of the on hand during the week for easy sandwiches. This low-carb bread recipe is ideal for meal prep and healthy lunchboxes.

With less than 6 grams of net carbs, over 40 grams of protein and 60 grams of fat, this meal is ideal for those who practice intermittent fasting and need a nutritious meal to break their fasting window.

Hands-on 10 minutes Overall 20 minutes

Ingredients (makes 1 serving)

1 Ultimate Keto Bun - see other suggestions below

1 small salmon fillet (115 g/ 4 oz)

1 tbsp avocado oil, olive oil or ghee (15 ml)

2 slices bacon (60 g/ 2.1 oz)

2 leaves lettuce (10 g/ 0.4 oz)

1 slice tomato (27 g/ 1 oz)

1 slice red onion (8 g/ 0.3 oz)

1 tbsp mayonnaise (15 g/ 0.5 oz) - you can make your own mayo

Note: Instead of keto buns, you can make a regular Keto Bread Loaf and slice to make a sandwich (flax-free and nut-free option included), or Nut-Free Keto Buns if you can't eat nuts.

Instructions

1) Preheat grill pan or skillet to high heat. Season the salmon with salt and pepper. Add the oil to the skillet then crisp up the bacon
2) Sear the salmon skin side down for 5 minutes until it easily releases from the pan. Flip and cook 2 more minutes. Remove and set aside.

3) To assemble, slice the bun in half and layer in the lettuce, salmon, onion, tomato, bacon, and mayonnaise.
4) Serve immediately.

Ingredient nutritional breakdown (per serving)

Net carbs	Protein	Fat	Calories
Ultimate Keto Buns, homemade			
4.3 g	10.1 g	15.9 g	208 kcal
Salmon, raw			

0 g	24.9 g	6.8 g	168 kcal

Avocado oil, extra virgin

0 g	0 g	14 g	124 kcal

Bacon, streaky (high fat content), organic

0 g	8.2 g	15.1 g	169 kcal

Lettuce, green leaf, raw

0.2 g	0.1 g	0 g	1 kcal

Tomatoes, fresh

0.7 g	0.2 g	0.1 g	5 kcal

Onion, red, fresh

0.5 g	0.1 g	0 g	3 kcal
Mayonnaise			
0.1 g	0.2 g	12.5 g	111 kcal
Total per serving			
5.8 g	43.8 g	64.3 g	789 kcal

Spicy Beef Keto Hot Pockets

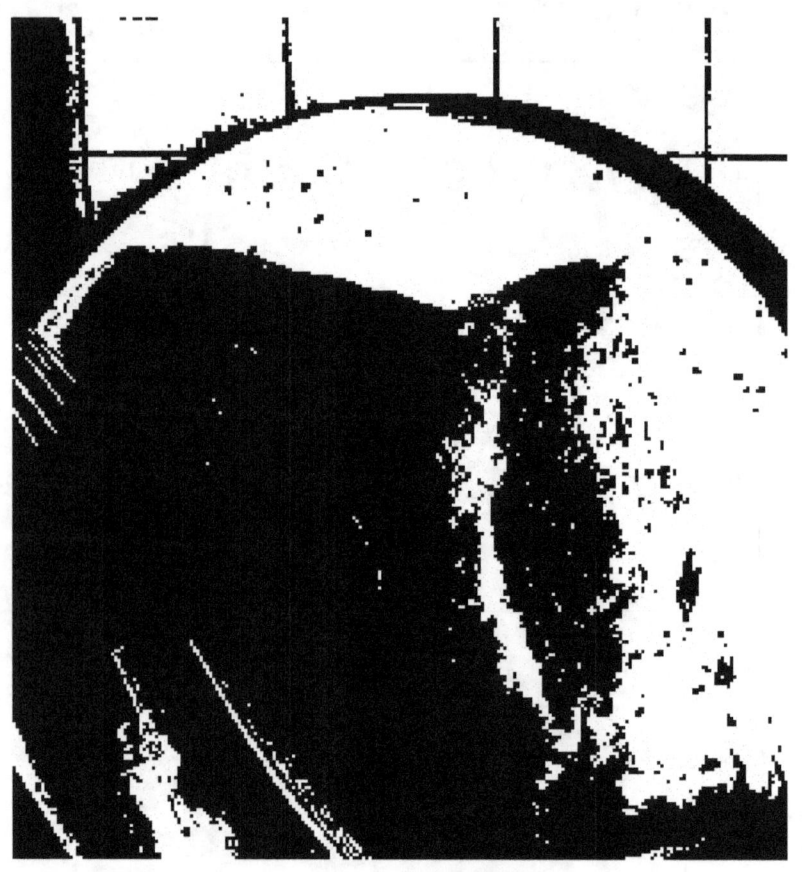

If you've not tried our Keto Hot
Pockets yet, you're in for a treat.
These spicy beef hot pockets are
packed full of flavour, not too hot but

if you're a chilli lover you can totally up the anti and go chilli mad.

I served these low-carb spicy beef hot pockets to Mr B (my food critic and chief taste tester) and I couldn't help but chuckle at the big thumbs up, you're through to the next round wave. He thinks he's John Torode off Masterchef! LOL!

These keto-friendly hot pockets make a great low carb lunch idea or comfort food dinner, served with a simple side salad.

Hands-on 15 minutes Overall 35 minutes

Ingredients (makes 2 servings)

Filling:

1/2 small brown onion (35 g/ 1.2 oz)

2 garlic cloves (6 g/ 0.4 oz)

1 tsp ghee or butter

300 g ground beef (10.6 oz)

1 - 2 small chile peppers, chopped (10 g/ 0.4 oz)

1 tsp coconut aminos

1 tsp Sriracha sauce (you can make your own Sriracha)

1/4 tsp sea salt, or to taste

1/4 tsp black pepper, or to taste

1 cup fresh spinach (30 g/ 1.1 oz)

Dough:

3/4 cup shredded low-moisture mozzarella (85 g/ 3 oz)

1/3 cup almond flour (33 g/ 1.2 oz)

Instructions

1) Preheat the oven to 200 °C/ 400 °F (conventional), or 180 °C/ 355 °F (fan assisted). Chop the onion and garlic. Heat the ghee in a non stick or cast iron pan on a medium heat.

2) Add the onion and fry for 2 minutes until soft. Add the garlic for a further 30 seconds. Add the

beef and cook for approximately 5 more minutes until cooked through, breaking the mince up with a spatular until fine.

3) Add the chilli, coconut aminos, sriracha and season to taste. Stir through the spinach, cooking for 1 - 2 minutes until wilted. Turn off the heat and place to one side.

4) Melt the mozzarella in a microwave for about 60 seconds until the mozzarella melts. Add the almond flour and mix to combine to form a dough.

5) Roll between two sheets of greaseproof paper or one sheet and a silicone mat.

6) Place the chilli beef mixture in the centre and fold to seal the dough.

7) Careful prick or slice a few air holes in the top.

8) Place on a greaseproof lined baking tray and bake in the oven for 15 - 20 minutes until golden.areful prick or slice a few air holes in the top.

9) Best served fresh - enjoy!

Ingredient nutritional breakdown (per serving)

Net carbs	Protein	Fat	Calories
Onion, brown (yellow), raw			

1 g	0.2 g	0 g	6 kcal

Garlic, fresh

0.9 g	0.2 g	0 g	4 kcal

Ghee

0 g	0 g	2.5 g	23 kcal

Beef, minced (ground), raw, grass-fed

0 g	25.8 g	30 g	381 kcal

Peppers, chile (chili), fresh

0.4 g	0.1 g	0 g	2 kcal

Coconut aminos (substitute to soy sauce)

0.2 g	0 g	0 g	1 kcal

Sriracha chili sauce, hot sauce

0.5 g	0 g	0 g	2 kcal

Salt, pink Himalayan rock salt

0 g	0 g	0 g	0 kcal

Pepper, black, spices

0.1 g	0 g	0 g	1 kcal
Spinach, raw			
0.2 g	0.4 g	0.1 g	3 kcal
Mozzarella cheese (low moisture, for pizza)			
2.4 g	10.1 g	8.4 g	125 kcal
Almond flour (blanched ground almonds, almond meal)			
1.5 g	3.6 g	8.8 g	98 kcal
Total per serving			
7.2 g	40.3 g	49.8 g	647 kcal

Easy Pork Chops With Asparagus and Hollandaise

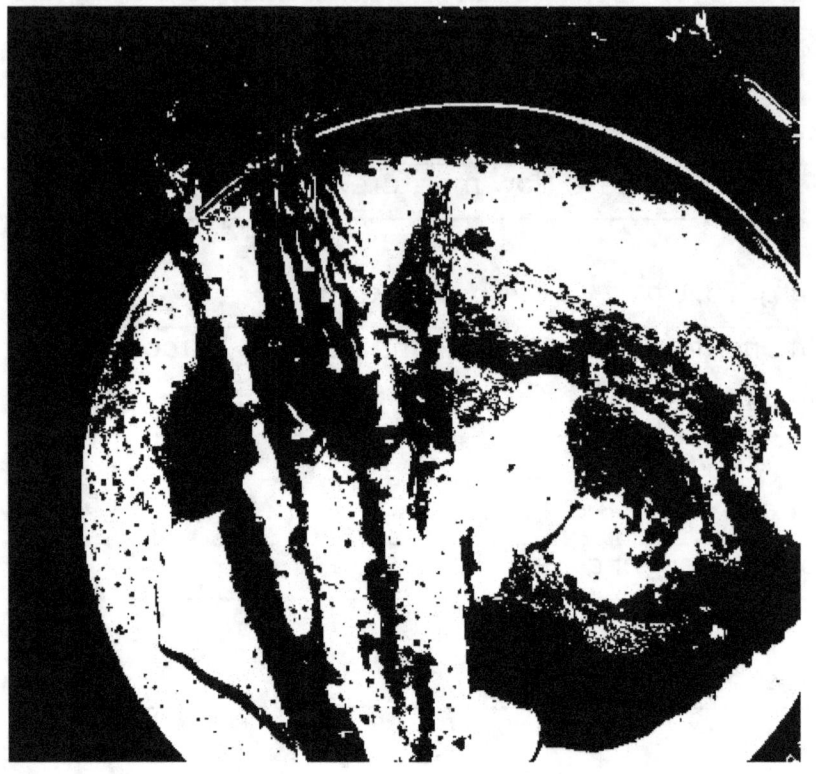

This is a quick and easy weeknight dinner.

Tender and juicy pork chops, teamed with sweet spears of asparagus, lovingly blanketed in the fastest hollandaise sauce you'll ever make.

At less than 3 grams of net carbs per serving, it's also perfect for those nights when you need a super low carb meal. Enjoy!

Hands-on 10 minutes Overall 20-25 minutes

Ingredients (makes 3 servings)

1/2 cup butter, ghee or extra virgin olive oil (120 ml/ 4 fl oz)

3 large egg yolks

1 tbsp lemon juice (15 ml)

3 pork loin chops, bone in (200 g/ 7.1 oz each), or use 3 boneless pork chops (150 g / 5.3 oz each)

2 tbsp ghee or lard (30 g/ 1.1 oz)

300 g asparagus spears (10.6 oz)

salt and pepper, to taste

Note: If a recipe calls for raw eggs and you are concerned about the potential risk of Salmonella, you can make it safe by using pasteurized eggs. To pasteurize eggs at home, simply pour enough water in a saucepan to cover the eggs. Heat to about 60 °C/ 140 °F. Using a spoon, slowly place the eggs into the saucepan. Keep the eggs in the water for about 3 minutes. This should be enough to pasteurize the eggs and kill any potential bacteria. Let the eggs cool down and store in the fridge for 6-8 weeks.

Instructions

1) Prepare the one-minute Hollandaise. Place 1/2 cup butter or ghee into a wide mouthed jar, with enough room for a hand blender to fit into. Melt the butter in the microwave.

2) Add the egg yolks and the lemon juice. Place the hand blender in the bottom of the jar and blitz until well combined, lifting it

slowly as you blend. Taste and season, if required.

3) Heat a frying pan over med-high heat and melt the remaining ghee. Cook the pork chops for 6 minutes on each side and then rest for 5 minutes.

4) Meanwhile, bring a pot of water to the boil and then blanch the asparagus for 5 minutes. Remove from the water and drain well.

5) Serve pork chops with asparagus spears placed over them, and then drizzle the hollandaise over the top.

6) Store the pork and asparagus in the refrigerator, wrapped for 2 days.

7) Store the hollandaise in its jar, with the lid on, in the refrigerator for 4 days, warming it before use.

Ingredient nutritional breakdown (per serving)			
Net carbs	Protein	Fat	Calories
Butter, unsalted, grass-fed			
0 g	0.3 g	30.7 g	271 kcal
Egg yolk, fresh			
0.6 g	2.7 g	4.5 g	55 kcal
Lemon juice, fresh			
0.3 g	0 g	0 g	1 kcal
Pork, chops (loin), boneless, raw			
0 g	30.7 g	13.4 g	252 kcal
Ghee			
0 g	0 g	10 g	91 kcal
Asparagus, fresh			
1.8 g	2.2 g	0.1 g	20 kcal
Salt, sea salt			

0 g	0 g	0 g	0 kcal

Pepper, black, spices

0.1 g	0 g	0 g	0 kcal

Total per serving

2.8 g	36 g	58.8 g	690 kcal

Keto Portobello Mushroom Mini Pizzas

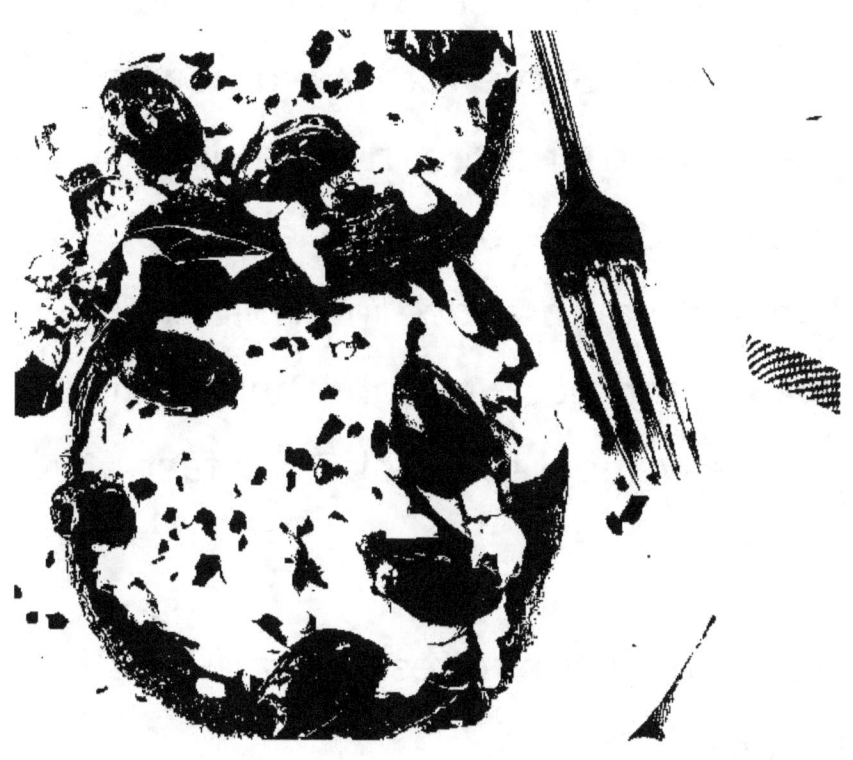

A fun and easy quick keto meal, these portobello mushroom pizzas will be a hit with the whole family!

This low-carb recipe is also a great way to add in a ton of vegetables to your diet while keeping your carb intake low. Serve with a big bowl of green salad dressed in olive oil or homemade mayo and it's a great option if you practice intermittent fasting and need a high-energy, quick and easy meal to break your fast.

Hands-on 10 minutes Overall 20-25 minutes

Ingredients (makes 2 servings)

2 large portobello caps, stems removed (170 g/ 6 oz)

1/2 cup pesto (125 g/ 4.4 oz) -you can make your own pesto

10 black kalamata olives (30 g/ 1.1 oz)

1 tbsp canned peppers (10 g/ 0.4 oz)

1 tbsp capers (9 g/ 0.3 oz)

1 cup shredded Italian blend cheese (115 g/ 4 oz)

Optional: pinch of crushed red pepper and basil for garnish

Note: Apart from olives, pickled peppers and capers, you can top these mini pizzas with chopped sun-dried tomatoes, green olives, chopped pepperoni or bacon. Instead of pesto you can use our homemade marinara sauce.

Instructions

1) Preheat oven to 190 °C/ 375 °F (conventional), or 170 °C/ 340 °F (fan assisted) and place the mushrooms on a baking sheet. Divide the pesto between the mushrooms. (You can reserve the portobello stems and add them on top of your breakfast omelet.)Tip for the perfect portobellos: Baked mushrooms can be watery. To reduce the moisture, brush the

portobellos with a small amount of ghee or olive oil and bake without the topping for 10-12 minutes. Add the topping and broil on high for another 2-3 minutes.

2) Fill the centers with the cheese then top with your desired toppings.

3) Bake for 10-15 minutes, just until the cheese is bubbly and the mushrooms are starting to soften.

4) Serve immediately, optionally sprinkled with red pepper flakes, or refrigerate for up to a day and reheat before serving.

Ingredient nutritional breakdown (per mini pizza)

	Net carbs	Protein	Fat	Calories
Portobello mushrooms, fresh	2.2 g	1.8 g	0.3 g	19 kcal
Basil & Macadamia Pesto (KetoDiet blog)	2.4 g	2 g	41.3 g	382 kcal
Kalamata olives	0 g	0.3 g	3.9 g	38 kcal
Peppers, sweet, green, canned, solids and liquids	0.1 g	0 g	0 g	1 kcal
Capers, canned				

0.1 g	0.1 g	0 g	1 kcal

ITALIAN 4-CHEESE BLEND, SHREDDED CHEESE

2 g	14.4 g	14.4 g	205 kcal

Total per mini pizza

6.8 g	18.6 g	60 g	646 kcal

Keto Salmon, Kale & Poached Egg Bowl

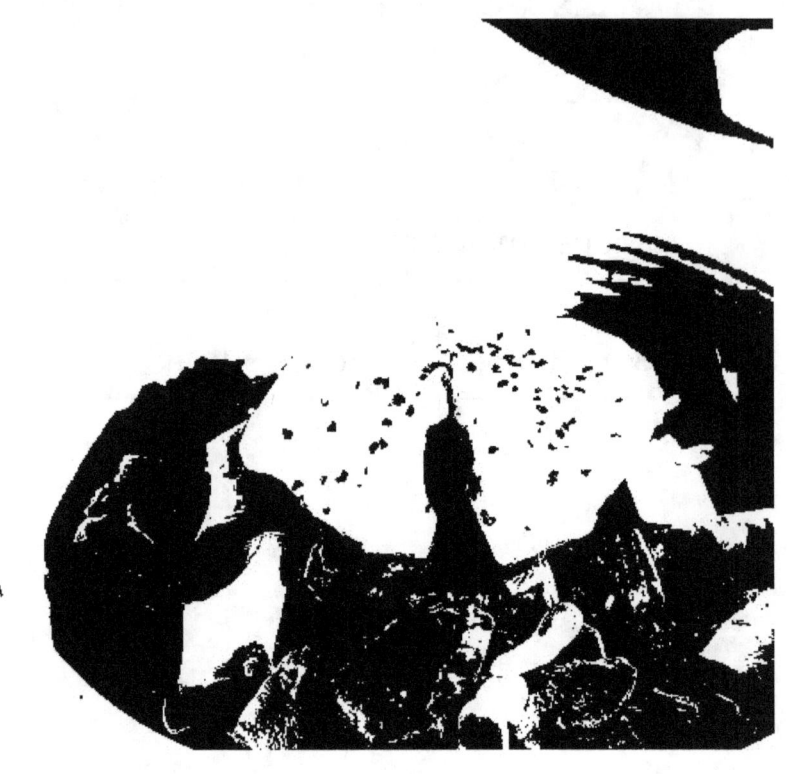

A breakfast, lunch or dinner favourite. Don't you just love a recipe that you fancy at any time of the day? This low carb roast salmon, kale and poached egg bowl is the perfect balance of healthy fats, fibre, carbs and protein to keep hunger at bay, insulin levels stable and your belly happy and healthy. It works really well with smoked salmon too if you prefer.

I used keto superfoods like salmon, avocado, kale and eggs. They are great sources of quality protein, healthy fats and electrolytes, making it the ideal dish for those who practice intermittent fasting while following a lchf diet. Whether you prefer skipping a meal or fast for

24 hours, this is the ideal low-carb recipe to break your fast.

Just one serving will provide over 70% of your daily potassium and 30% magnesium. And remember, if you just started following a ketogenic diet, don't be afraid to use salt. Sufficient sodium will keep keto-flu at bay!

Hands-on 20 minutes Overall 20 minutes

Ingredients (makes 2 servings)

3 1/2 cups curly kale (175 g/ 6.2 oz)

1 tbsp coconut aminos (15 ml)

2 tbsp extra virgin olive oil (30 ml)

2 tbsp toasted sesame oil (30 ml)

1 tbsp fresh lemon juice (15 ml)

pinch of sea salt and pepper

2 wild salmon fillets (300 g/ 10.6 oz)

1 tbsp ghee, butter or coconut oil (15 g/ 0.5 oz)

1 garlic clove, minced

2 large eggs

1 avocado, sliced (200 g/ 7.1 oz)

2 tbsp almond flakes

Instructions

1) Preheat the oven to 180 °C/ 355 °F (fan assisted). Mix the coconut aminos, olive and sesame oil, lemon juice, salt and pepper in a bowl.

2) Blitz or finely chop the kale. Massage the dressing into the kale and allow to stand whilst you make the salmon and eggs.

3) Heat the butter or coconut oil in a non-stick frying pan. Fry the salmon fillets, skin side up on a medium heat for about 3 - 4 minutes. Flip and cook for a further 3 minutes until cooked through.

4) Add the chopped garlic for the remaining 30 seconds – 1 minute until crisp. Remove the salmon from the pan and allow to cool slightly.

5) Place the almonds on a baking tray and roast for 6 minutes until golden. Remove from the oven and allow to cool.

6) Place a pan on water with a pinch of salt on the hob and bring to the boil. Crack the eggs separately into a cup. Swirl the water in a circular direction and gently pour in the eggs one at a time. Cook for 3 - 4 minutes on a medium heat for a medium poach (firm

white, runny yolk) or to your liking. Remove from the water and drain on kitchen roll.

7) Remove the skin from the salmon and pull into flakes.

8) Place the kale in a bowl, top with salmon and garlic, almonds, sliced avocado and perfect poached egg. Eat immediately.

Ingredient nutritional breakdown (per serving)

	Net carbs	Protein	Fat	Calories
Kale, curly, fresh	3.2 g	1.7 g	0.4 g	25 kcal
Coconut aminos (substitute to soy sauce)	0.5 g	0 g	0 g	2 kcal
Olive oil, extra virgin	0 g	0 g	13.5 g	119 kcal
Sesame oil	0 g	0 g	13.6 g	120 kcal
Lemon juice, fresh	0.4 g	0 g	0 g	1 kcal
Salt, sea salt				

0 g	0 g	0 g	0 kcal

Pepper, black, spices

0 g	0 g	0 g	0 kcal

Salmon, raw

0 g	32.4 g	8.9 g	219 kcal

Ghee

0 g	0 g	7.5 g	68 kcal

Garlic, fresh

0.5 g	0.1 g	0 g	2 kcal

Eggs, free-range or organic

0.4 g	6.3 g	4.8 g	72 kcal

Avocado, fresh

1.8 g	2 g	14.7 g	160 kcal

Almonds, nuts (flaked)

0.4 g	1.5 g	3.4 g	38 kcal

Total per serving		
7.2 g 44 g 66.6 g	826 kca	

Low-Carb Butternut Squash Lasagna

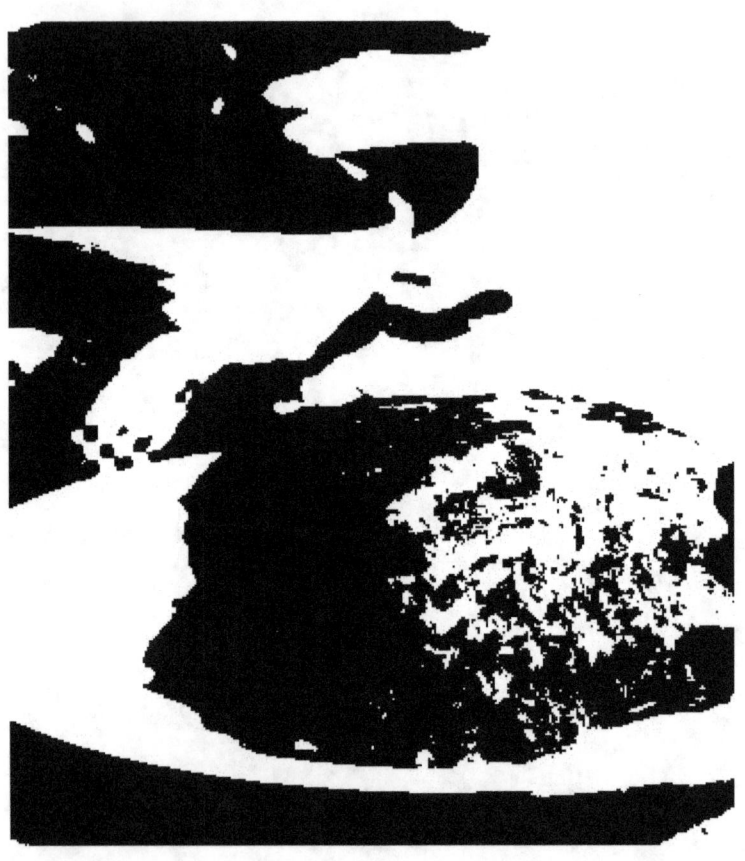

Comfort food doesn't get more classic than lasagne. My low-carb and gluten-free take on this Italian classic features delicious layers of thinly sliced butternut squash, homemade marinara sauce, ground beef, creamy herb-infused ricotta, melty mozzarella and crispy Parmesan.

I used pre-cut butternut squash from a local grocery store. If you can get pre-cut squash, it will save you a ton of time but if not, simply use a mandolin.

Although this grain-free lasagna is not ultra low in carbs, it can be included on a keto diet as long as you stay within your macros. It's high in nutrients and ideal for intermittent fasting when you eat one or two meals per day.

Hands-on 25 minutes Overall 1 hour 30 minutes

Ingredients (makes 6 servings)

1 batch Homemade Marinara Sauce (300 g/ 10.6 oz)

400 g butternut squash, thinly sliced (14.1 oz)

1 tbsp ghee or extra virgin olive oil (15 g/ 1.1 oz)

700 g ground beef (1.5 lb)

1 tsp dried oregano

1/2 sea salt or pink Himalayan salt

1/4 tsp black pepper

2 packs ricotta cheese (500 g/ 1.1 lb)

2 large eggs

2 tbsp chopped fresh parsley

2 tbsp chopped fresh basil

2 cups shredded mozzarella cheese (226 g/ 8 oz)

1/2 cup grated Parmesan cheese (45 g/ 1.6 oz)

Instructions

1) Prepare the Marinara Sauce by following this recipe. Preheat the oven to 200 °C/ 400 °F.

2)I used pre-cut butternut squash lasagne sheets. If you can't get pre-cut slices, simply peel the butternut squash and remove the seeds. Then use a mandolin to slice it thinly (about 1/8 inch or 1/4 cm).

3)Grease a large pan with ghee and add the ground beef. Cook for 5-7 minutes while stirring, or until opaque. Add half of the marinara sauce and oregano. Season with half of the salt and pepper.

4)Prepare the ricotta layer. Combine the ricotta, eggs, chopped parsley and basil. Season with the remaining salt and pepper.

5) Spread the remaining marinara sauce on the bottom of a large casserole dish. I used a 26 x 18 x 6.5 cm (10 x 7 x 2.5 inch) casserole dish. Add the first layer of butternut squash slices. You will use a total of 3 butternut squash layers.

6) Top with half of the ground meat mixture and half of the ricotta cheese mixture.

7) Add another layer of butternut squash slices and top with the remaining ground beef.

8) Spread the remaining ricotta cheese mixture on top of the ground beef.

9) Top with the remaining butternut slices, grated mozzarella and Parmesan cheese.

10) Cover the casserole with a baking foil and transfer into the oven. Bake for 45 minutes. Remove the foil and bake for 7-10 minutes.

11) Remove the lasagna from the oven and let it rest for 15 minutes before slicing. Once cooled, it can be stored in the fridge for up to 4 days.

Ingredient nutritional breakdown (per serving)

Net carbs	Protein	Fat	Calories
Marinara sauce			
2.2 g	0.6 g	8.2 g	84 kcal
Squash, winter, butternut or coquina			
6.5 g	0.7 g	0.1 g	30 kcal
Ghee			
0 g	0 g	2.5 g	23 kcal
Beef, minced (ground), raw, grass-fed			
0 g	20 g	23.3 g	296 kcal
Oregano, dried			
0.1 g	0 g	0 g	1 kcal
Salt, pink Himalayan rock salt			
0 g	0 g	0 g	0 kcal
Pepper, black, spices			
0 g	0 g	0 g	0 kcal

Ricotta cheese, full-fat			
2.5 g 9.4 g 10.8 g		145 kcal	
Eggs, free-range or organic			
0.1 g 2.1 g 1.6 g 24 kcal			
Parsley, fresh (spices)			
0 g 0 g 0 g 0 kcal			
Basil, fresh			
0 g 0.1 g 0 g 0 kcal			
Mozzarella cheese (low moisture, for pizza)			
2.1 g 8.9 g 7.5 g 111 kcal			
Parmesan cheese			
0.2 g 2.7 g 1.9 g 29 kcal			
Total per serving			
13.8 g	44.5 g	55.9 g	745 kcal

Low-Carb Beef Stew with Herby Dumplings

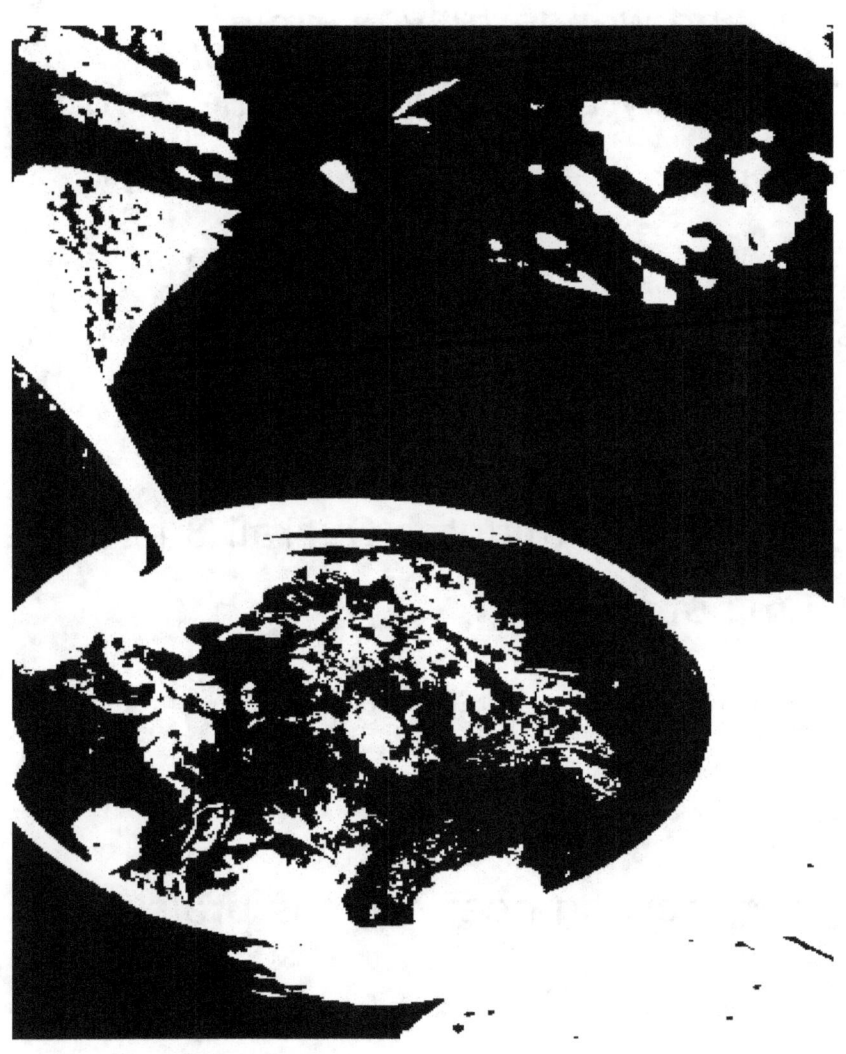

This braised beef stew is like your slouch jumper of Winter. Comforting, cosy and wonderfully warming. Gorgeously tender, melt in the mouth beef packed with lots of chunky low carb veg all bubbling happily in a sauce quite frankly I want to drink!

Hands-on 40 minutes Overall 3 hours 15 minutes

Ingredients (makes 6 servings)

Stew:

900 g stewing beef such as braising steak (2 lb)

2 tbsp extra virgin olive oil or ghee

1 medium red onion, chopped (100 g/ 3.5 oz)

200 g pumpkin, ideally Hokkaido (7.1 oz)

1 medium carrot (60 g/ 2.1 oz)

3 bay leaves

3 sprigs of fresh rosemary

2 cloves garlic, minced

2 tbsp tomato puree (30 g/ 1.1 oz)

1/2 cup dry red wine (120 ml/ 4 fl oz)

2 cups beef stock or beef bone broth (480 ml/ 16 fl oz) - you can make your own

3/4 tsp sea salt or pink Himalayan salt, or to taste

1/4 tsp cracked black pepper

Dumplings (makes 12):

3 large egg whites

1 large egg

1 cup water, boiling (240 ml/ 8 fl oz)

3/4 cup almond flour (75 g/ oz)

1/3 cup sesame seed flour (30 g/ 1.1 oz)

1/4 cup coconut flour (30 g/ 1.1 oz)

2 1/2 tbsp psyllium husk powder (20 g/ oz)

1 1/2 tsp gluten-free baking powder

1/4 tsp pink Himalayan or sea salt

1 tbsp chopped rosemary

1 tbsp fresh thyme

To serve:

1 tsp fresh lemon zest (about 1/2 lemon)

pinch cracked black pepper

fresh parsley for topping

Tips for Crockpot:

You can make this meal in your slow cooker. To do that, use just half of the stock in the stew and cook on low for 8 hours, or on high for 4 hours. Browning the meat prior to slow cooking is optional but highly recommended as it will enhance the flavour. Serve with the prepared keto

dumplings or with Cauli-Mash or
Celeriac Cauli-Mash.

Instructions

1) Preheat the oven to 160 °C/ 320
°F (fan assisted). Heat 1
tablespoon of olive oil in a large
pan. Brown the meat on a
medium heat for 5 minutes, stirring regularly to seal the meat for
approximately 5 minutes. Turn off
the heat and place to one side.
2) Meanwhile, peel the onion,
pumpkin and carrots and chop

into chunks about 2 cm (1 inch). In another pan heat one tablespoon of olive oil and fry the vegetables on a medium heat for 10 minutes, stirring regularly to prevent sticking.

3) Add the beef, rosemary, bay leaves, chopped garlic and tomato puree. Sauté for a further 2 minutes.

4) Add the red wine, reduce the heat and simmer for 5 minutes. Add the stock, season with salt and pepper, bring to the boil.

5) Place a casserole dish in the oven to heat up. Place the stew in the casserole dish and add a lid. Roast in the oven for 3 hours until

the meat is tender and the juices have concentrated. Remove from the oven once cooked. Turn up the oven to 175 °C/ 350 °F.

6) Make the dumplings as per the keto bread recipe 1. Grease a cupcake tin with olive oil to prevent sticking. Shape into dumpling shapes (3 to 4 cm/ up to 1-1/2 inch in diameter) and place individually in the cupcake holes. Bake in the oven for 25 minutes. Turn over with a spoon and place back in the oven to cook for a further 5 minutes.

7) Place the stew back in the oven to heat through if cooled slightly. Add the dumplings.

8) To serve, place the stew in bowls and top with grated lemon zest, fresh parsley and a pinch of cracked black pepper.

9) Apart from dumplings, you can serve this stew with Cauli-Mash or Celeriac Cauli-Mash!

Ingredient nutritional breakdown (per serving, stew + 2 dumplings)

Net carbs	Protein	Fat	Calories
Beef (for slow cooking), grass-fed			
0 g	28.8 g	27 g	366 kcal
Olive oil, extra virgin			
0 g	0 g	4.5 g	40 kcal
Onion, red, fresh			

1.1 g	0.2 g	0 g	7 kcal

Squash, Hokkaido, raw

2.3 g	0.4 g	0 g	10 kcal

Carrot, fresh

0.7 g	0.1 g	0 g	4 kcal

Bay leaf, dried

0.2 g	0 g	0 g	2 kcal

Rosemary, fresh

0.1 g	0 g	0 g	1 kcal

Garlic, fresh

0.3 g	0.1 g	0 g	1 kcal

Tomato purée (paste, unsweetened)

0.4 g	0.1 g	0 g	2 kcal

Red wine (dry)

0.5 g	0 g	0 g	16 kcal

Beef bone broth

0.2 g	1.2 g	1 g	13 kcal

Salt, pink Himalayan rock salt

0 g	0 g	0 g	0 kcal

Pepper, black, spices

0 g	0 g	0 g	0 kcal

Egg white, fresh

0.1 g	1.8 g	0 g	9 kcal

Eggs, free-range or organic

0.1 g	1 g	0.8 g	12 kcal

Water, still

0 g	0 g	0 g	0 kcal

Almond flour (blanched ground almonds, almond meal)

1.1 g	2.7 g	6.6 g	74 kcal

Sesame flour, fine, defatted

0.3 g	2.3 g	1 g	20 kcal

Coconut flour, organic

0.5 g	0.9 g	0.8 g	18 kcal

Psyllium husk powder

0.3 g	0.1 g	0 g	2 kcal

Baking powder, gluten-free

0.3 g	0 g	0 g	1 kcal

Salt, pink Himalayan rock salt

0 g	0 g	0 g	0 kcal

Rosemary, fresh

0 g	0 g	0 g	0 kcal

Thyme, fresh

0 g	0 g	0 g	1 kcal

Lemon zest (peel), fresh

0 g	0 g	0 g	0 kcal

Pepper, black, spices

0 g	0 g	0 g	0 kcal

Parsley, fresh (spices)

0 g	0 g	0 g	0 kcal

Total per serving, stew + 2 dumplings

8.5 g	39.8 g	41.8 g	599 kcal

...gramcontent.com/pod-product-compliance
... Source LLC
...burg PA
...31280526
...0001B/130